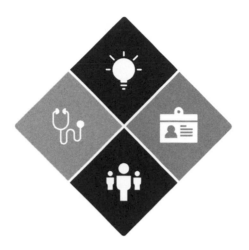

THE **E** FACTOR

How Engaged Patients, Clinicians, Leaders,
and Employees Will *Transform Healthcare*

CRAIG DEAO, MHA

Published by:
Fire Starter Publishing
350 West Cedar Street
Suite 300
Pensacola, FL 32502
Phone: 866-354-3473
Fax: 850-332-5117
www.firestarterpublishing.com

ISBN: 978-1-62218-080-6

Library of Congress Control Number: 2016962906

The stories in this book are true. However, some names and identifying details have been changed to protect the privacy of all concerned.

Printed in the United States of America

To the team who cared for my father-in-law and the millions of caregivers around the world just like them. You make lives better.

TABLE OF CONTENTS

FOREWORD

We each got into healthcare to make a difference in the lives of others. As healthcare providers, the most fulfilling days are realized when patients are engaged with their own health and with their caregivers. The more we focus on helping others engage, the more we engage ourselves.

All kinds of market forces are converging to create urgency for engagement. There's the industry move to preventative care under population health, a slew of financial incentive programs by CMS, and savvy new competitors—like CVS MinuteClinics—entering the market. And that's just a few for starters. Never have the stakes been so high.

At Studer Group®, we know that to be the trusted advisor for organizations to build a culture of high engagement is both a great privilege and a great responsibility. It starts with leading by example. That's why we're committed to creating a work environment that fosters high engagement. Year-over-year, our employee engagement ranks in the 99th percentile.

How do we do it? Engagement starts at the top with maintaining transparent and open communication, setting clear expectations, building trust, and requiring personal accountability. What do employees need to engage? They want and need to feel a sense of purpose, that they're doing worthwhile work, and that they are making a difference. They want and need to feel valued and to have good relationships with their leaders. They want opportunities for professional development and career advancement.

Craig Deao's passion for this work leaps off of these pages. It furthers our mission—to make healthcare better for employees to work, physicians to practice medicine, and patients to receive care. His breadth and depth of knowledge is backed by years of research, development, and coaching. He knows that change and excellence are achieved when we commit to doing the *right thing, every time*. His expertise has proven time and again how Evidence-Based Leadership^SM fuels engagement, and ultimately the flame for this sacred work we do. I'm grateful to Craig for his exemplary leadership and the time and dedication he has put into sharing his learnings with us all.

Debbie Ritchie, President
Studer Group

INTRODUCTION

In December 2014, my father-in-law was diagnosed with a four-centimeter glioblastoma. It was devastating news to hear about a man who had never skipped work due to illness during his 47 years of employment. Aureliano "Jaime" Ruiz had been the picture of health.

When he got the diagnosis, he'd recently celebrated his 50th wedding anniversary with my mother-in-law, Mari. A close-knit family, they'd raised their children in Mexico, later moved to Sterling, Illinois, in the 1970s, and were just now beginning to enjoy their retirement together.

It was during that anniversary celebration—the summer of the World Cup, in fact—that I watched 77-year-old Jaime outmaneuver my boys, who were five and seven years old then, in a game of soccer. As a professional soccer player in his youth, he had a strategic advantage that compensated for the years as he used his cane to knock soccer balls out of the corner of the goal. It was unbelievable!

So you can imagine our shock when this man—whose only experience with healthcare was an emergency appendectomy—was diagnosed with a brain tumor. His prognosis was even more shocking: just two to three months to live. With surgery, radiation, and chemotherapy, we were told, his life could possibly be extended nine to twelve months.

Jaime told his kids while growing up that you've got to fight for what you want. My wife remembers a picture of him that her sister proudly displays on her refrigerator: He's got his fists up, always reminding us to give it everything we've got.

And fight he did. Even though he was terrified of surgery, he decided it was his best chance to spend more time with his family. Unfortunately, it did not go well. Soon after the surgery, we moved him to an inpatient rehabilitation facility in El Paso where he lived, in the hope that he could regain some strength post-op to prepare for radiation and chemotherapy.

During those dark days—the 70 days from when he was diagnosed until his death just two days shy of his birthday, on February 19, 2015 —Julie traveled from our home in Pensacola, Florida, to El Paso, Texas, to be with her father as part of the care team. Many of us in healthcare have been in that role, not only as a caretaker but also as part of the healthcare team. It's the role you never wanted, but the one your family needs from you nonetheless. If you haven't had this experience, chances are good that one day you will.

As you can imagine, during those days, Julie and I shared a lot of tears on the phone. She missed the boys, was grateful to be with her family, experienced continuous fear and anxiety, and was truly exhausted. But Jaime was never left alone, not during post-op, hospital stays, inpatient rehab, or even in hospice. Mari, Julie, or one of her siblings was always with him.

There were also moments of shared relief and comfort during that tough time. The most remarkable of these were because of some simple, yet powerful experiences at Highlands Rehabilitation Hospital. Jaime and his family had an exceptional experience with the care team there.

As luck would have it, our organization had just begun coaching Highlands as part of our partnership with their system, Vibra Healthcare. In fact, I was scheduled to speak to a roomful of CEOs from across their 30+ long-term acute care hospitals in a few weeks' time. The Highlands CEO would be among them.

So I encouraged Julie to write a letter I could read to them about what was so special at Highlands; her letter became a case study of what engagement looks like through the eyes of a family member.

Julie began by telling me about Travis. She said, "Dad experienced anxiety with new caregivers, but when Travis came into the room he gave my dad confidence that nothing would happen to him while he was on duty. When another caregiver accidentally hit the code blue button, Travis sprinted into the room. We didn't know what was wrong, but he said he wanted to attend to Dad quickly because, 'I care for your dad as if he were *my* dad.'"

My wife, who had been in healthcare for 15 years prior to our move to Florida, can quickly sort through genuine concern and canned bravado. Travis's words made a difference.

She told me about Manny. During Jaime's stay in the ICU, he had delusions at times, making it difficult to sort through what was real and what was not. Jaime began to believe he'd won the lottery. In fact, he believed this so fervently that he asked Julie to write Manny a check for a million dollars.

Why Manny? Because Manny spoke to him in Spanish, his preferred language. And mostly, because during a transfer at the hospital, a young aide almost dropped Jaime, which made him anxious about transfers after that. Manny created a lighthearted mood while transferring Jaime, talking and joking with him in Spanish. He also called him "Mr. Jimmy," unaware that it was a term of endearment used by his brothers. What a difference a couple of words meant.

Julie explained that her dad was also very modest, but he allowed Manny to shower and bathe him, even at his most vulnerable. It was all about *trust*. And that simple act of respect built trust. Trust builds engagement. And engagement, as you'll read, unlocks everything.

She told me about Sharna, who was so professional. "She made Dad feel confident in her abilities by always telling him what she was going to do before she did it, when she was going to do it, and why he needed to take each medicine."

She told me about Gus, Estella, Jennifer, and Frank, who also made a difference for Julie and her dad. She mentioned Maria, one of the nurses on duty when her dad coded and was rushed to the ED in the middle of the night for both a heart attack and a lower GI bleed. He was frightened and helpless. But Maria stayed by his side, held his hand, and—for the moments before the ambulance took him—whispered over and over, "You're going to be all right." And he was that night.

There was Victor, who sat down with Julie and her family and shared his own personal family loss. He showed them true, authentic empathy.

And then there was Dr. Eric Spier, the first doctor among the many he had seen who took time to sit in front of Julie's dad, rather than stand. Dr. Spier addressed Jaime directly, rather than only his family who were sitting around the table, even though Jaime was so weak that he was dozing off. Julie conveyed how appreciative they were of that simple act. After all, it was his illness, not theirs.

He invited Julie to attend the team meeting, where he addressed all of her concerns regarding her dad's future and asked her input about what she was seeing when the care team wasn't in the room. He was the only doctor who shared the news they had known but just hadn't heard yet from anyone on the care team. It takes courage to tell a family that any additional treatments may not extend the quality of life for the person they love.

Julie sums up the team by explaining that "Dad's biggest loss was his independence. The indignity of having other people bathe you, stick you, feed you, keep you alive when your body and your mind betray you is devastating. These people gave him back some level of respect by being compassionate, kind, and honest, and he appreciated that." And so do I.

I didn't get to meet this team. But I was blown away when Helen Carmona, the CEO at the hospital, attended Jaime's wake and his funeral, along with some of her colleagues. Julie's family and her mom were so touched. Who wouldn't be?

I know this genuinely caring behavior wasn't a fluke. In most hospitals and doctor's offices, most of the time, our caregivers and leaders do amazing things like this. It's happening right now. Tens of thousands of caregivers— right now as you read this—are choosing to say or do something with a patient and family member because they know it's the right thing to do. Even though no one is watching. Even though it's not going to be documented in the chart or earn additional reimbursement. They're doing it because that's what engaged professionals do.

I also know it's not just about the caregivers. There can't be a care team without a patient and, at times, their family. Julie and her family asked questions. Uncomfortable questions. They sought second opinions and also made decisions as members of the care team, rather than passively accepting what the doctors said. Julie also committed to giving feedback...some of it was positive feedback, like the letter I was able to read that day, and some of it was uncomfortable, constructive feedback...and no doubt hard to hear.

At Studer Group®, a Huron solution, we know that even when the outcome isn't what we want, we can still create an exceptional experience for patients and families. After all, patients and families routinely rate their experiences with hospice care as outstanding.

The key question is how do we move from *most* of the time in *most* places for *most* patients to *always*? The answer—just as it always is when we talk about high reliability and reducing variation in any practice—is that leaders make the difference.

If we want caregivers to engage with their patients, then leaders need to create an environment where they can practice the kind of medicine or nursing or therapy that motivated them to get into their profession in the first place. And to achieve that, we must relentlessly improve the systems and processes that surround the care team, ensuring they have what they need to do the job and removing those obstacles that get in the way and erode the joy we all need to feel to do our best work.

I'll be sharing more about what this engagement model looks like in upcoming chapters. Essentially, leaders create an environment in which caregivers can be perpetually engaged. Caregivers create an environment that facilitates engagement by patients. And when patients are engaged? Well, that's where the magic is. It's why I wrote this book.

At Studer Group, our mission has always been to create better places for employees to work, physicians to practice medicine, and patients to receive care. We're passionate in our belief that when we engage these three key stakeholders, we unlock the strategic advantage that separates healthcare from every other industry: our people. The evidence is clear that if we can maximize human potential, we achieve our shared mission of making healthcare better.

And that's the goal of this book: to help you understand what engagement is; how to foster it; and what works to create the highly engaged leaders, employees, clinicians, and patients who will transform healthcare into the system we all need it to become.

PART ONE

Why Is Engagement So Crucial?

Twenty years ago, this book would have focused on the term *satisfaction*. Back then, it was the best measure we had to understand the viewpoints of our employees, physicians, and patients. But today, most healthcare leaders have shifted their employee and physician measures toward *engagement*, recognizing the strong connection between engagement and other key metrics such as productivity and quality.

What do we mean by *engagement*? It's much more than satisfaction or happiness. In the case of an employee, it's about being emotionally invested in and focused on creating value for the organization and the patient every day. Think about this simple example: If I want to leave work two hours early and my supervisor approves, I'm satisfied, right? But how engaged am I in the pursuit of that organization's mission in those two hours? Not at all. I can be satisfied, yet not engaged.

While satisfaction is a one-way street ("What's the organization doing for me? What do I get?"), engagement is a two-way street ("How are we partnering together to create value?"). It's about giving discretionary effort, even when no one is watching. It's about tapping into that reservoir to decide if I— as an employee, a clinician, or a patient—will decide to take a specific action or not. Engagement means closing the "knowing-doing" gap so that a person has more than the right plan…they actually get it done.[1]

Now it's time to embrace patient *engagement*, just as we've done with our employees and physicians. As an industry, we've expanded our thinking about how patients perceive their care by including measures of experience alongside the traditional measures of satisfaction, giving us additional insight that strongly links to quality and safety. Yet neither satisfaction nor experience is quite the same as engagement.

While there is no widely accepted definition of patient engagement, the concept is that patients are actively involved in the process of care—in terms of processing information, deciding how care fits in their lives, and acting on those decisions.[2]

But to get engaged patients, we need engaged clinicians and employees. So the question becomes: How engaged are these stakeholders who are so crucial? Sadly, not as engaged as we need them to be. Research shows that worldwide, only 13 percent of workers are engaged. We fare a bit better in the United States with 30 percent of Americans engaged in their jobs.[3]

But still, that means that *70 percent of people who show up for work are not engaged.* How can we hope to achieve our mission and vision without the other 70 percent?

The benefits of engaged employees and physicians have been well documented. Patient engagement is a more recent area of research, but the emerging picture is impressive. In short, engaging patients is the most effective way to achieve our big aims in healthcare: to dramatically reduce cost while improving quality.

Engaged patients strive to be informed about their health, are involved in healthcare decisions, and participate in self-care. They assume responsibility and accountability for the role their behaviors play in their care outcomes. They self-monitor and provide information; they offer feedback on their experience and outcomes, and commit to making long-term lifestyle changes. They take greater responsibility for their health, which may be the single biggest lever we have for improving outcomes and reducing costs in healthcare today.

However, the sad reality is that patients are not sufficiently engaged. Consider the facts: 40 percent of deaths today are caused by modifiable behavioral issues.[4] Unfortunately, changing those behaviors typically requires upfront costs in time, money, and commitment for an individual to reap long-term rewards. But we often discount those future rewards because the present looms larger…leading to good intentions that end in procrastination and lack of follow-through.[5] Habits are hard to change.

People with chronic diseases take only 50 percent of prescribed doses…and just 50 percent of patients follow referral advice.[6] In addition, fully 75 percent of patients do not keep their follow-up appointments![7] One of the most frustrating results when patients aren't engaged manifests in what is often referred to as "medication non-adherence."

I recently heard a remarkable statistic showing the magnitude of this issue. In one 2008 study, more than 3 percent of prescriptions were filled by the pharmacist but never picked up by the patient.[8] If this so-called "prescription abandonment" rate holds true for the 3.6 billion prescriptions filled in pharmacies that year, it means that 110 million prescriptions were actually abandoned in 2008. Of course, that doesn't even take into account the large percentage of patients who begin to take a prescription—say, an antibiotic—but stop when they feel better in three days and never finish the prescribed 10-day course.

It's easy to see why highly engaged patients are so crucial in healthcare today; we can't fix the healthcare cost crisis without them. Chronic diseases, like diabetes and cardiovascular diseases, account for the majority of deaths and more than 75 percent of the nation's medical care costs.[9]

The challenge, of course, is that the average patient visit with a clinician lasts just 20 minutes, and the average patient sees a doctor just three times per year. In other words, he spends just *one* hour per year with the doctor. *What about the other 8,764 hours?* Those 20 minutes will need to influence the next 2,921 hours before the next visit.

This is where the idea of accountable care comes in. While we typically think about the accountability the hospital and the doctor have under emerging reimbursement models, accountable care also requires the *patient* to be accountable. Think about it: Chronic diseases like diabetes and cardiovascular disease are largely preventable. There are three key behaviors that have a significant impact: (1) increasing physical activity, (2) controlling weight, and (3) quitting smoking.

If we want to motivate patients to take responsibility for shifting their health during the many hours we aren't seeing them, we need to create environments that facilitate their engagement, helping shift the paradigm from "the doctor will fix me" to "I'll get the support I need to take charge of my own health." But here's the thing: Research and experience show that patients will engage at this level only through an authentic partnership with their caregivers.

If we want patients to take responsibility for their health, we must empower, motivate, and inform them by facilitating a sense of connection and trust and by using a team approach with communication and other types of tools that make it easy to demonstrate our steadfast commitment to their success.

To achieve that, we will need to count on highly engaged caregivers and healthcare employees. There's just no substitute for engaged stakeholders; it's the holy grail for transforming our industry…the key to delivering on our promise of higher clinical quality at a lower cost.

Let's talk next about what else is driving the need for engagement in healthcare today.

CHAPTER 1

Engagement Isn't Optional
(The Transformation of Healthcare Depends on It!)

Let's begin with an honest look at the state of our industry. First, the good news: Healthcare has recruited the best and the brightest from across the land. If you think about the kids who are in classrooms today—the ones getting the top test scores, working for extra credit, those who demonstrate passion, curiosity, and creativity every day—those are the ones who are disproportionately attracted to a profession in healthcare.

Just think about the physicians you know. Sure, they could've taken their great intellect and applied it to advancing research, working in the lab every day, but they decided instead to apply what they've learned in the interest of helping other people. Even those of us who aren't clinicians, but work in healthcare delivery...we want to have purposeful, worthwhile work that makes a difference.

That's good news for engagement: If you can connect the actions you're asking people to take to their core values, they'll commit to doing them. And commitment is a much better outcome than mere compliance. It's the advantage we have over many other industries, because if we can leverage that talent and maximize its potential—which is exactly how we express our vision at Studer Group®, by the way—then we can accomplish anything.

Physicians Aren't Just Disengaged—They're Burned Out

When it comes to doctors, healthcare is in the midst of a burnout epidemic. In his book *Healing Physician Burnout*, Quint Studer notes that 30 to 65 percent of physicians are burned out.[1] This can vary by specialty, but in some specialties, it's as many as one in two physicians.

What do we mean by physician burnout? They are emotionally exhausted; they have compassion fatigue; and they've lost confidence that they can be effective due to a whole slew of challenges and obstacles that impact their perceived ability to provide high-quality care to their patients.

But to realize a culture of high engagement, we desperately need engaged physicians. If you think about it, the opposite of burnout is really just being neutral. But that's not good enough. We need to move them all the way up to highly engaged.

Why? We know that engaged physicians deliver better health and steward resources more effectively. One example: When a physician actually discusses smoking cessation, patients are about 30 percent more likely to quit smoking.[2] That's a 30 percent improvement just because a physician has a conversation!

Studies also show that engaged physicians deliver 51 percent more inpatient referrals, are 26 percent more productive, and bring in $460,000 more annual patient revenue.[3] In other words, engaged physicians are crucial to both clinical outcomes *and* healthcare operations. So we have to address this issue of burnout before we can even approach engagement.

Satisfaction Is Necessary, But Insufficient

In healthcare, we've measured satisfaction for a long time…employee satisfaction, physician satisfaction, and patient satisfaction. And it's important to understand satisfaction levels. It's necessary, but it's also not enough.

Some organizations have found ways to bump up satisfaction levels by letting employees dress more casually or by valet parking patient cars in a crowded parking lot. And, while those are nice things that do increase satisfaction, it's just not the same as creating *engagement*.

It's not enough to just be present. In fact, there's a term that human resources executives have coined more recently called "presenteeism" that takes the concept of "absenteeism" to the next level. We know absenteeism is a problem; when our employees don't come to work, they obviously can't be engaged in the work we do. But presenteeism describes someone who comes to work, and yet isn't engaged. *Harvard Business Review* defines it as "at work, but out of it."[4]

Perhaps an employee is sick and is technically sitting in her chair, but she's not feeling well enough to be meaningfully attending to her work; or, maybe she is perfectly healthy and has a great attendance record, but hates her job and needs the money so she wastes a lot of time.

In any case, make no mistake about it: Presenteeism has real costs in the workplace. Consider the reduced productivity of workers in pain, for example. Two articles in the *Journal of the American Medical Association* report that depression costs U.S. employers $35 billion in lower performance,[5] and back problems cost nearly $47 billion.[6] The point is that employees who are physically present at work isn't enough. We need them to be highly engaged in advancing our mission, vision, and values on a daily basis.

When it comes to patients, the healthcare industry has made a big shift toward measuring patient experience over the past 10 years. While experience shouldn't replace satisfaction as a single patient-reported measure, it does add more dimensions. And perhaps most importantly, it allows us to measure patients' perception about very specific aspects of quality.

In other words, if you look at the various surveys used by the Centers for Medicare & Medicaid Services (CMS), they're not asking if a patient is satisfied or dissatisfied. The questions ask, "Did you never, sometimes, usually, or always" observe some evidence-based practice happening. That's a frequency survey, not a satisfaction survey.

The survey wants to know to what degree you as a patient understood the side effects of medication, how often your pain was controlled, and to what degree you received information that you would need to care for yourself after discharge. Essentially, "How often did you see a specific evidence-based practice that correlates with quality happen at the bedside?"

These questions identify valid quality issues and offer real evidence of our industry moving toward patient-centered care…because no industry gets to define quality without listening to the voice of their customer. It's no different from when you buy a new car and are asked to share your perception of your customer experience.

Why Engagement Matters, Now More Than Ever Before

Industry dynamics and market forces are now combining to create an unprecedented level of industry change…all signaling new urgency for a culture of high engagement. To meet those challenges successfully will require us to take the next leap forward.

There's no question that patient engagement is gaining traction as a key success factor in healthcare reform. Clearly, there is consensus among stakeholders that patient engagement is a high priority for meeting goals laid out in the Affordable Care Act. In fact, the ACA's Preventable Readmissions Program aims to reduce the estimated $1.7 billion spent on readmissions.[7]

Because engagement directly impacts quality, there are a number of new strategies shaping healthcare reform with this focus. These range from programs like the Institute for Healthcare Improvement's Triple Aim to CMS's Quality Strategy.

Additionally, the industry's seeing more partnerships by stakeholders, like Robert Wood Johnson's Aligning Forces for Quality and the CMS-sponsored Partnership for Patients, which aims to reduce preventable hospital-acquired conditions by 40 percent.

Engagement is also front and center today in federal programs that qualify organizations through financial incentives, most notably CMS's rule for meaningful use, which is designed to increase patient engagement, and CMS's Medicare Access and CHIP Reauthorization Act of 2015 (MACRA), which transitions providers to a new Medicare payment model, at least partly dependent on certain patient engagement and access competencies.

What else is driving the shift to engagement in healthcare today? Competition from other industries. Healthcare is facing new pressures to better engage its customers due to the threat of losing them to new competitors—retailers and technology companies among them—from other markets. CVS is a prime example, a company using its core competency to meet customer needs fast and conveniently, to now compete with primary care providers through its MinuteClinics.

In addition to all these incentives for high engagement, a number of market forces are converging that also make patient engagement a high priority. Due to the rapid advances of biomedical research and precision health, for example, we can anticipate over the next five to fifteen years that we will have a much deeper understanding of how an individual—based on their DNA, genetic make-up, and other health factors we can measure—will respond to certain treatments…and perhaps even how to keep individuals healthier longer.

The era of targeted, predictive, and personalized medicine is here. Meanwhile, sensor technology continues to explode, both in terms of speed and portability, just as our ability to meaningfully tap into big data accelerates, for lightning fast analysis of health patterns and trends.

A quick example of what this looks like: Recently, at a meeting I attended, one of the individuals in our group woke up not feeling well, complaining of a fast heart rate. Another colleague—who happened to be a cardiologist—opened an app on his phone called Kardia (which bills itself as "proactive heart health") and proceeded to place the thumbs of the person with the fast heart rate on two little metal boxes—about the size of two postage stamps—located on the bottom of his phone. He then hit the button on the app and got an instant EKG trace that is medically accurate.

Now, because he's a cardiologist, he could read that EKG directly, but for $2, you or I could request that a board-certified cardiologist read and interpret it. Next, he converted the EKG to a PDF and emailed it to her. Because he suspected something was going on, he urged her to head to the emergency department, where she shared that EKG and was admitted to the hospital for overnight observation.

You can begin to imagine a very different type of customer experience in healthcare in the years to come, both in terms of how we think about our health as individuals and in how we will consume care. Millennials who are infinitely comfortable with technology will likely expect their clinicians to be highly engaged with their care on a real-time basis.

The question is: What are we doing to prepare our organizations *today* to harness the power of these trends and engage with consumers in a meaningful way? The one-time transactional relationships that have often characterized acute care in the past will fade away as we increasingly find ways to personalize care quickly with ongoing connectivity and two-way dialogue over the long-term.

If our goal is to improve the patient experience, however, this is all good news. Frequent touchpoints and long-term connectivity are likely some of the best ways to encourage customer loyalty over a lifetime.

Another force creating pressure for engagement is patients themselves. The stark reality is that employers have shifted the cost of care to consumers through high-deductible plans. As a result, consumers are becoming more cost conscious and are demanding more transparency about costs as they comparison shop, requiring healthcare providers to adjust the way they allocate costs. They're also more likely to check what their insurance covers when choosing tests and treatments. And yet, few health plans offer cost and quality information to help them make informed decisions.

The Kaiser Family Foundation reports that average annual out-of-pocket costs have risen nearly 230 percent per employee between 2006 and 2015.[8] As consumers feel this increasing cost pressure, they are hungry for information on how to make better healthcare decisions.

In some ways, this higher level of engagement by consumers clearly aligns behaviors to reduce costs. One 2013 study showed that nearly half of patients in high-deductible plans chose a generic instead of a brand-name drug and one-third asked about alternative treatment options and costs.[9]

Unfortunately, an important and unintended negative consequence of shifting the financial burden to consumers is that patients are forgoing medical care—tests, treatments, follow-up appointments, and drugs—due to high costs. A 2015 Gallup study found that just shy of 31 percent—almost one in three Americans—have delayed medical treatment because of the cost.[10] Even as far back as 2009, a Thomson Reuters study of 12,000 households found that 21 percent of people surveyed were delaying or postponing care because it wasn't affordable.

And, the problem gets worse if you consider low or middle income patients as they did in one study that found that these individuals—the very population for whom we are trying to improve access to healthcare in this country— were more likely to forgo or defer care.[11] In fact, this same study found that it's a vicious cycle: Doctors of individuals who haven't had regular medical care typically order more tests and treatments, which creates a greater financial burden, which in turn leads to patients who don't follow doctors' orders, which then sustains poor health.

But isn't the whole point of the Affordable Care Act to improve access to care for this population? you might ask. Let's take a quick look at that. It turns out that 62 percent of consumers who selected one of the plans available through the healthcare exchanges chose the bronze plan with a family deductible of greater than $10,000.[12] So a large majority is essentially buying catastrophic health insurance.

If we then add the cost of the annual family premium, that family will assume $18,000 in costs to access healthcare. If we consider that the median household income in the United States is $53,657, that means that fully 33 percent—one-third—of that family's income is potentially going toward payment of healthcare costs.[13] Is that a sustainable proposition?

In one 2014 study, three out of five U.S. bankruptcies were predicted to be a result of medical bills.[14] You can begin to see the massive scale of financial stress American families are experiencing today with respect to healthcare costs. Increasingly, some forward-thinking health systems are responding with proactive solutions to consumer cost issues that threaten to derail the patient experience and make bad debt unmanageable. Engagement is the name of the game.

For one thing, providers are redesigning the revenue cycle to talk about costs and payment plans on the front end of care (rather than after the fact), offering financial counseling *before* treatment and procedures. In their quest to meet their mission for healthy communities, some organizations are also responding to the affordability crisis by proactively discounting charges or offering charity care to patients with much higher incomes than in the past.

It's All about Value

When we think back to all those government and quality initiatives we examined a few pages back, what's the point really? It's value. Value-based care is about delivering higher quality for a lower cost. Accountable care organizations, meaningful use regulations, new reimbursement formulas...they are all designed to provide more value for patients and those who foot the bill. And really, transformation of the healthcare industry in this respect is no different from any other industry. There's upward pressure on quality and downward pressure on price.

Think about the last time you bought a laptop or other computer. Was it faster than the one you replaced? Undoubtedly. If it follows Moore's Law, the processing power, a dimension of quality, is literally twice as fast.

Now think about what you paid for that new laptop. You probably paid the same, or even less. You got higher quality for a lower cost. And, like with the computer industry, that's what has occurred in the steel manufacturing industry in the 1980s. It's what has happened to automobiles and televisions. And it's happening today in healthcare, too.

As a result, incentives are steering patients to organizations that produce the best value: the highest quality at the best prices. In addition to improving value, our industry is also trying to reduce that other V word: variation. Because even in organizations that typically provide high quality at a low price, there is still extraordinary variation.

Variation isn't acceptable. It's not enough to deliver *most* of the time. That's why CMS's CAHPS surveys today ask about *always*. They want to see a culture of *always* and have developed reimbursement formulas that reward for that. An *always* culture requires commitment—not compliance—from the people doing the job to do it right. Every time. And it requires engaging the customer in a whole new experience too.

> ### An *always* culture requires commitment from the people doing the job to do it right. Every time.

Just think about the banking industry for a moment. It's an industry that underwent a consumer-centric revolution to deliver higher quality. Remember bankers' hours? That whole concept is extinct. Today, banks offer 24/7 banking from any smartphone. You or I could withdraw our money from an ATM in Bangladesh tomorrow if we wanted to. It's a completely different way of thinking about the role the customer plays and how we must redesign our business practices around those needs. That's the shift the healthcare industry is undergoing today.

Plus, population health is coming...and relationships make all the difference. As reimbursement models continue to shift away from fee-for-service and increasingly toward payment systems where providers agree to total spending targets for certain populations of patients, patient engagement becomes critical to reengineering care successfully to meet all of our goals. You can't manage the health of a population without their involvement in self-management.

It's Time to Take Action

So in summary, all these market forces and trends in healthcare are combining to create a new imperative for engagement. It's time to take action. If we want to achieve all those big aims we've been discussing—improving clinical outcomes with a better patient experience at a lower cost—engagement is a prerequisite.

Sure, the healthcare delivery system needs to hold itself accountable for its part in reigning in our ever-escalating costs. We're too expensive, and that's not even examining the role of the pharmaceutical industry or insurers in their contribution to the cost crisis. They have a role to play, too.

But by far, the biggest costs we need to address —about 75 percent of costs— are those posed by the cost of managing chronic diseases, as we have discussed. And those are precisely the costs that can be most impacted by highly engaged patients.

How will we get there? The good news is that we know what works. Studer Group's evidence-based methodologies—and the coaches who provide them—have earned a reputation for how to build, benchmark, and sustain cultural transformation, precisely because we know how to nimbly apply "simple-to-understand-but-hard-to-execute" strategies that effectively engage people. If you're familiar with Studer Group's work, you'll find that the tools we'll share in upcoming chapters are familiar, but have been adapted for engagement.

Even before Studer Group began its journey to receive the 2010 Malcolm Baldrige National Quality Award, our success with "people systems" was well established. The company has been named seven times consecutively to the top 10 list of best places to work among small to medium companies by Great Place to Work®, the global authority on building, sustaining, and recognizing high-trust cultures. A decade of employee engagement surveys consistently places Studer Group in the top 1 percent of more than 500 similar businesses.

But one of the things we learned in our journey to becoming Baldrige-worthy was that in our quest for world-class outcomes, we had built a people-centric business along with a process-loving culture. Baldrige showed us that it takes more than hiring A+ talent to win the Olympics; you have to also create and refine A+ systems and processes...so that even C-level talent can get Olympic-level results. Of course, when you hire A+ talent and pair it with A+ systems and processes—with a commitment to continual improvement—that's when you truly sustain world-class Olympic-level excellence.

If you've been on the journey to performance improvement in recent years, you already understand how employees and physicians drive organizational performance through high engagement. Now, it's time for the final piece: engaged patients.

Key Learning Points: Engagement Isn't Optional

1. Engaged patients realize better clinical outcomes at a lower cost.

2. Engaged patients are those who strive to be informed about their health, are involved in healthcare decisions, and participate in self-care.

3. Satisfaction is necessary but insufficient.

4. Industry dynamics and market forces are now combining to create unprecedented change in healthcare. These all signal new urgency for a culture of high engagement to effectively transform our industry and deliver on our promise of value-based care.

5. The good news is that we know what works. Evidence-Based Leadership[SM] methodologies that have proven to increase employee, physician, and patient satisfaction and patient experience can be successfully adapted to improve engagement, too.

CHAPTER 2

Engagement Is a Comprehensive Strategy

Human behavior is still the biggest source of variance when it comes to health-related outcomes, despite the huge advances technology has delivered.[1] What people do, or don't do, will ultimately determine a great deal of our long-term health.

And it's not just about the patients' choices and actions. Clinicians and leaders can highly influence engagement, so their actions are also critical. That's why we need to consider engagement a core organizational competency; it has a direct and positive impact on reducing this variance.

Engagement needs to be a visible strategy within the organization—one that is both intensive and comprehensive—because this idea of connecting or not connecting truly touches every interaction. It's the glue that holds our culture together.

Think for a moment about how we talk about patients who don't follow physician advice. When they don't take their medications as prescribed or follow through with medical recommendations, we often label them as "noncompliant." At times, it's even noted in a patient's chart, which then brands that patient as "difficult" or "troublesome" for the next physician interaction. Labels can stick.[2] Remember—words matter when it comes to engagement.

What does "non-compliance" really mean, anyway? Dr. John Steiner, a researcher at Kaiser Permanente in Colorado suggests that the idea of non-compliance by patients is a gross oversimplification. In a recent article, he imagined a patient in his late 60s with diabetes, hypertension, and high cholesterol and tallied up everything that patient would need to do to be considered compliant with all medical recommendations.[3]

It added up to more than 3,000 annual behaviors, which ranged from filling and refilling five different prescriptions and complying with dietary recommendations to getting regular exercise and blood tests before every appointment. That's a lot to ask of a human being.

That's why it's so important for clinicians to be empathetic to patients and to help them identify and resolve barriers that get in the way of following through on recommendations. And that type of sensitivity training can start right in medical school.

To help her medical students understand this challenge firsthand, Dr. Ofri, an associate professor of medicine at New York University School of Medicine, wrote up prescriptions for a number of medications: metformin, Lasix, albuterol, lisinopril, and ranitidine.

Next, she handed each student two prescriptions and two boxes of Tic Tacs as substitutes for the actual medicines, with the instructions to take the "medicines" for a week. The next time they met, not one of the students said they were able to take every single pill as directed for seven days.[4] Clearly, it's easier to write out a prescription and a few recommendations for patients than it is to actually follow them.

What Do We Really Know about the Patients We Want to Engage?

Today, the average electronic health record is awash in clinical and financial data, but doesn't tell us much specifically about the person being treated. This isn't a new problem. For 30 years, patients have been complaining about repeating the same information multiple times in the same system.

We are still missing some of the most useful information to create engagement. For instance: What motivates that individual? What influences and guides his personal decision making process? How will these influences impact his treatment and willingness to follow his physician's care plan? This is the kind of information that can facilitate *engagement*.

Let's dig a little deeper as we consider some of the critical information that is missing about our patients today and the resulting consequences. If a hypothetical patient John Bell lives in the city, but doesn't drive, and his physician refers him to a specialist in the suburbs, he's likely to be a no show...which then leaves that physician idle, that appointment unavailable for someone else, and the patient unable to benefit from the visit.

But if instead, the physician and his office team know Mr. Bell doesn't drive, they could refer him to a specialist close to public transportation, or arrange for transportation. The chances that he will keep the appointment increase dramatically.

In the same way, if Mrs. Otillio cares for her husband at home with a chronic illness, she may be reluctant to leave him to pick up her prescription at a pharmacy. (One of those cases of "prescription abandonment" I mentioned earlier.) But if her physician knew in advance that she was in a caregiver role, and arranged for her prescription to be delivered to her home or ensured she left with the prescription in hand, she would be far more likely to take her medication as prescribed.

When it comes to reducing hospital readmissions, knowing more about our patients and acting accordingly can have a big impact as well. For example, just knowing whether a patient has a friend or family member who lives close by to help with post-discharge recovery could be vital. In fact, it turns out that whether that friend or relative lives within 10 miles can be a significant predictor of readmissions.[5]

If we want patients to truly engage in their health and wellness, it's important to understand their personal health goals, not those "prescribed" by the physician, but the quality of life an individual ultimately wants to achieve.

That's why it's so important to have the right tools and structure to truly make it easy for patients...a knowledge-based infrastructure that drives workflows, clinical decisions, and clinical directives to truly address the personal motivations of patients to achieve their personal goals.

However, when it comes to talking about "non-compliance" or "non-adherence" at Studer Group®, we prefer to focus on gaining a patient's "commitment" to the role they play as part of the care team. *Committed* patients better represent an agreement about our shared values and a partnership, while compliance is really about fulfilling basic, perfunctory responsibilities.

> ***Committed* patients better represent an agreement about our shared values and a partnership, while compliance is really about fulfilling basic, perfunctory responsibilities.**

We're interested in a higher order. Just as we do with employees and clinicians, we're looking for commitment from patients. And the best way to facilitate that is if every interaction patients have within our organization demonstrates engagement.

Engagement Must Become a Core Organizational Competency

When I think about organizations that really live the principles of engagement every day, I inevitably think of Advocate Good Samaritan Hospital in Downers Grove, IL.

"We understand we're primarily in the relationship business," CEO Dave Fox explains. "We believe relationships are the gateway to accomplishment." He takes this thought even a bit deeper when he echoes the ancient Chinese philosopher Lao Tzu: "The way to do is to be."

The idea is that engagement is much more than a list of "to-dos." An effective engagement strategy has to start with a leadership culture that promotes an authentic attitude toward doing what's right for doctors, nurses, employees, and ultimately, patients. It's a way to "be."

Fox says that in Western cultures, there's often an attitude of "do" first, so we can then "have," and eventually "be" (i.e., "If we use a new communication tool, then our HCAHPS scores will be better, so our reimbursement will be higher.") But in Asian cultures, they recognize the "being" part must come before "doing," so we can then "have" (i.e., "If we feel care and compassion for our patients, then our employees will want to use new communication tools that drive better clinical outcomes. Their values will compel it!")

When your values compel you to do the right thing, engagement is inevitable. For example, as someone who grew up with a general surgeon for a father, Dave Fox is particularly sensitive to the burdens, responsibilities, and, also, the nobility, of physicians' work. And he's stayed close to those values.

In fact, in his very first week as new CEO at Advocate Good Samaritan back in 2003, he demonstrated this priority to physicians when, at a two-hour physician-hospital board meeting, he agreed to refund $950,000 to the struggling physician-hospital organization to improve their economic situation.

He did this even though he had to immediately call the chairman of the board and explain he'd just given away 10 percent of the hospital's net budgeted income for the year. He explained that it was the right thing to do; he recognized that the hospital's success is dependent on physicians' success and he wanted to demonstrate that to them. Today, physician engagement at Advocate Good Samaritan is top-notch.

Context is everything. How do you get this "being" thing right? Fox says, "You have to provide explicit context for everything you're trying to do by connecting back to the underlying purpose, vision, and values that drive each of us in healthcare. The bigger the context for what we want people to do, the bigger the outcome is going to be."

In his book *The Heart of Change*, management guru John Kotter shares the idea that you can't change behavior through logic; rather, you change it by touching people's hearts and emotions. Kotter says, "Changing behavior is less a matter of giving people analysis to influence their thoughts than helping them to see a truth to influence their feelings."[6]

Imagine that you, as CEO, need to communicate a reduction in workforce at your next all-staff meeting. On the one hand, you could take the victim approach by saying, "As you know, healthcare reform is coming. Reimbursement just isn't keeping up with inflation, so times are tougher now. We're going to be forced to lay off 200 people over the next month just to survive."

Or, you could create context that aligns with your vision and values by explaining, "Healthcare is becoming unaffordable for people. As a result, we and other healthcare organizations need to move from a fee-for-service model to a population health model, where our job will be to keep people well and out of the hospital...so we can reserve the hospital for patients who are truly sick."

You might continue by explaining, "Making healthcare easier and more affordable is the right thing to do. But there are challenges. It means we will be reducing our length of stay and admissions. While we are still trying to grow market share, we do need to manage down the size of the workforce. Our plan is to find jobs for anyone who is displaced and also to begin by no longer filling positions that are now vacant."

Which approach would be more likely to motivate you more as an employee in that room? When transparency aligns with our values, we create trust, the very foundation for fostering relationships, alignment, and, ultimately, engagement. Without that trust, you can be busy rolling out new tools and tactics that no one ever embraces. And we all know that the problem with evidence-based tactics is that they work only if people actually do them!

When transparency aligns with our values, we create trust, the very foundation for fostering relationships, alignment, and, ultimately, engagement.

Engagement is really about organizational *transformation*; it's much more than just change. Change is about doing or having something better or different with what is already possible or already exists. Transformation, on the other hand, is about doing what is *not* currently possible, unless or until you change how you are *being*.[7]

A comprehensive approach to engagement means you feel it everywhere at every level in the organization. For example, when you walk through the door at Advocate Good Samaritan Hospital, you'll see a prominent sign on the front door that reads, "Welcome to this place of healing."

It's a patient promise that Fox circles back to with staff and clinicians regularly in his communication to ensure the organization delivers. "If relationships are the foundation for a core competency of engagement, then communication is the action of leadership," he adds. "Communication isn't complete until an audience understands, embraces, and ultimately owns the message. We can never over-communicate."

Clearly, it's working. A winner of the Malcolm Baldrige National Quality Award, the hospital has been ranked in the top 100 U.S. hospitals by Truven Health Analytics for six consecutive years now and has been recognized as a Leapfrog A-rated hospital since the inception of that recognition. With a current serious safety event rate at 0.86 safety events per 10,000 adjusted patient days, the organization is on a journey to get to zero by 2020.

There are many examples of others, in addition to Advocate Good Samaritan, that excel at engagement as a core competency. If you think about companies like Nordstrom, USAA, or Southwest Airlines, they consistently demonstrate an incredible connection between the way they engage their employees and customers that translates into better outcomes, both in terms of the quality of the service or product they provide and their financial successes.

It's the same in healthcare. If you want highly engaged and loyal patients and family members—individuals who participate as active members of the care team and are accountable for their outcomes—then you need to have highly engaged and loyal clinicians who practice the kind of bedside care that facilitates engagement even when no one's watching, the kind of care that continues to have a positive impact on the patient's engagement as a member of the care team even between visits.

Engagement Is a Higher Order than Satisfaction

Earlier, I talked a bit about how satisfaction is necessary, but insufficient. It's clear that higher patient satisfaction is meaningful to improving the quality of the care we provide and building loyal relationships with patients. In fact, Studer Group first helped to put patient satisfaction on the CEO's to-do list almost 20 years ago now. Back then, it was the only measure we had. And it's still vitally important.

But since those days, we've learned about dramatic differences between what the terms patient *satisfaction* and patient *experience* mean. And yet, the practices that we can use to influence patient experience aren't vastly different from those for satisfaction; we just need to adapt them. Key words are helpful for both, for example, but we might choose different words. Clinical processes also needed to be adapted to address aspects of the patient experience that go beyond satisfaction.

What's important to recognize here is that we didn't move away from the idea of satisfaction; we added to it. In other words, while a patient might have been happy and satisfied with care, the actual bedside experience is what is most likely to correlate with the quality and safety outcomes to which we aspire.

When we consider patient experience, we are asking patients *how frequently they observed evidence-based practices* that correlate with better quality occur while they received care. Engagement is about whether they're going to take action and change their own behaviors. While both are important, they are clearly distinct measures.[8]

> **Engagement is about whether patients are going to take action and change their own behaviors.**

Consider, for a moment, a personal healthcare experience that you enjoyed recently. Did you feel nurtured? Did your clinician demonstrate compassion? Was everything easy? You likely felt satisfied.

The good news is that because you were satisfied, you were more motivated and likely to commit to actively participating in your care. When our psychological emotional needs are met as patients, it's conducive to our higher engagement. It's important to remember that patients don't necessarily seek to engage during healthcare encounters, but do respond when the conditions are right.[9]

Think of satisfaction as one of three components of engagement. To be engaged, you first need to be satisfied; you also need to feel that you can be effective, and you need to be motivated. Satisfaction is a prerequisite for engagement.

Satisfaction is a prerequisite for engagement.

Over the past decade, Studer Group has coached organizations to embrace a comprehensive shift to support engagement as an essential competency across all stakeholders. In the 1990s, we talked about employee satisfaction and physician satisfaction as a means to patient satisfaction. Today, Studer Group partner organizations are working toward employee and physician engagement as a means to gain patient engagement. The stakeholders remain the same.

If You Can't Measure It, You Can't Manage It

It's a classic business maxim you're likely familiar with. Just as organizations have learned to measure satisfaction and patient experience to drive action planning for improvement, it's important the healthcare industry begin to consider ways to measure engagement.

At the forefront of this effort is Dr. Judith Hibbard, a professor emerita at the University of Oregon and chief researcher at Insignia Health, the company now offering patient activation surveys based on her work. Hibbard's research team created a measure called the Patient Activation Measure—or PAM scale—that assesses patients based on 10 (or 13) questions about their personal experience, skills, knowledge, and commitment to make lifestyle changes. And it seems to be gaining traction. In fact, in June 2016, the

National Quality Forum endorsed this measure as a patient- and family-centered care measure.[10]

Hibbard defines patient activation as "the patient's knowledge, skills, ability, and willingness to manage his own health and care" and assigns "four distinct activation levels with specific needs, goals, and approaches to move the patient toward self-directed management."[11]

This definition of activation is an apt way of describing the "knowing-doing" gap I referenced in Chapter 1. (If five frogs are on a lily pad and one decides to jump, how many frogs remain on the lily pad? The Answer: all five of them. Deciding and jumping is *not* the same thing.)

It's true that activation and engagement differ. Just as a satisfied employee may not be an engaged employee, an activated patient may not yet be an engaged patient. Hibbard's patient activation assessments gauge the state of what's in someone's head by scoring them on their level of agreement or disagreement with certain statements (i.e., "I am confident I can tell a doctor my concerns, even when he or she does not ask," or, "I know what each of my prescribed medications does").

Based on their responses, patients are scored on a 0 to 100 scale. The score can be used to sort patients into four categories or "levels of activation," where the lowest level (level one) describes a patient with a very passive approach to his healthcare, and the highest level (level four) describes a patient with a proactive approach to partnering in healthcare.

As a result, PAM scores represent an important and foundational tool to assess patient readiness for engagement. Let's look at two significant findings from Hibbard's early research. First, patients with the lowest activation have the most expensive costs, and vice versa.[12] Here's what that looks like:

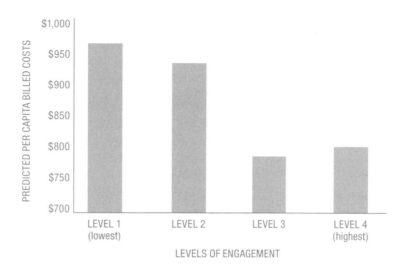

Figure 2.1 | **Actively engaged patients have lower costs.**

Source: Data adapted from Hibbard, Greene, and Overton 2013, 216-222.

Note: Demographics and clinical risk score were controlled variables.

In another study of Boston patients co-authored by Hibbard, researchers found that readmissions were twice as high for the least engaged patients compared to the most engaged patients.[13] Equally important, her research team identified that highly engaged patients are more likely to perform exactly the kinds of health-improving behaviors that correlate with better outcomes, from managing their cholesterol and not smoking to taking advantage of preventative screenings that allow for early detection and appropriate use of the emergency department.[14]

It makes intuitive sense, doesn't it? When a patient with congestive heart failure actually makes efforts to modify his lifestyle after a hospital visit, he is less likely to be readmitted and more likely to have a better outcome.

But engagement not only improves readmissions; more engaged patients also manage HDL and triglycerides better, are less likely to smoke and be obese, are more likely to get pap smears and mammograms, manage depression more appropriately, and they have fewer ED visits and hospitalizations.[15] Engagement is a powerful tool for health outcomes. Take a look:

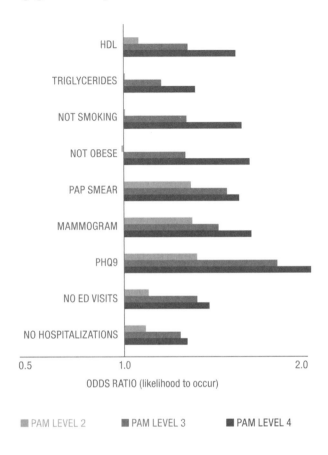

Figure 2.2 | Actively engaged patients have better outcomes.

Source: Data adapted from Greene et al, "When Patient Activation Levels Change,
Health Outcomes and Costs Change Too," Health Affairs, March 2015.

Note: Predicted outcomes two years after baseline PAM measurement.

"When it comes to activation, it's about supporting a patient's skill development and competence," explains Dr. Hibbard. "The goal is to create an environment so that patients can do for themselves because we've helped them acquire the skills they need to succeed." In other words, engagement is not some type of intervention with a patient.

We can't *make* them become activated; we can only make the conditions ripe for activation. And of course, we all know this from our own life experience; you can't change anyone. But you can create an environment that supports them so it is easier to make those changes.

We want to create an environment where that's *convenient* and *likely*...where the best choice is the easiest choice. It's very similar to the idea behind auto-enrollment in a company 401(k) plan. If we enroll employees automatically in the plan, but allow them to opt out, more employees will grow their savings by default.

There are even examples of this in healthcare today. In one study, researchers found that long-acting but reversible methods of contraception were almost 22 percent more effective than "refillable" methods, like birth control pills and patches.[16] Why? It's easy, convenient, and likely to continue once the initial decision has been made, much like the 401(k) automatic enrollment scenario above.

There are important implications with respect to Dr. Hibbard's research. For one thing, PAM scores tend to correlate with patient satisfaction; when you compare patients with high and low PAM scores who have seen the same physician, the patients with higher PAM scores are more satisfied, probably because they better understand their personal role in wellness and how to more effectively get the resources they need from the health system. Studies also show that patients with lower PAM scores are more likely to report poor care coordination, probably because passive patients are more apt to feel disappointed.[17]

Also, guess which patients tend to take advantage of online portals or resources for chronic disease self-management? Activated patients. If that's all your organization is doing to engage patients, you're likely missing the patients you need to engage most...those with low PAM scores. It will take more active outreach and attention to reach those.

Engagement Is a Cascade

We've already touched on the fact that if we want engaged and loyal patients, we must find a way to engage employees and clinicians first. At its core, engagement is about trust.

How can we convince patients to trust us? We use a suite of evidence-based communication tools. For example, key words, like AIDET Plus the Promise[SM], keep patients informed, reduce anxiety, and manage up our skills and experience. I'll share more about these tools on building trust in upcoming chapters.

But to ensure consistent use of these tools with patients, we'll need engaged clinicians and employees. That kind of engagement depends on hiring the right individuals, training them, and holding them accountable...which requires engaged leaders.

In short, engaged leaders create environments that allow clinicians to become engaged, who in turn commit to the type of patient interactions that facilitate engaged patients. It's a cascade of engagement.

> **Engaged leaders create environments that allow clinicians to become engaged, who in turn commit to the type of patient interactions that facilitate engaged patients. It's a cascade of engagement.**

As you can see in this model below, everyone who works in healthcare either cares for patients directly or cares for those who care for patients. No one is exempt from engagement.

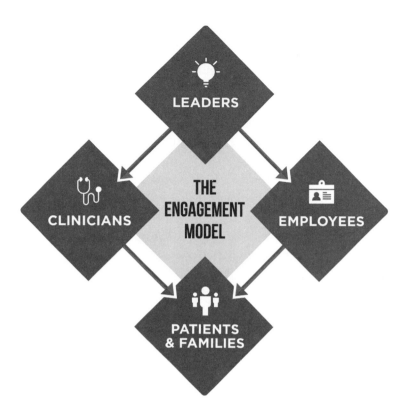

Figure 2.3 | Engagement flows from leaders to clinicians and employees and then to patients and families.

Sometimes at Studer Group we coach organizations that are physically located just down the block from each other, where one organization has high employee and physician engagement and the other is really struggling. Both organizations share the same payer mix and the same workforce pool. The difference? Leadership.

Trust starts at the top of an organization. It's leaders who are responsible for providing an environment for the care team to be focused on caring for patients with moments of communication and empathy, without systems and processes getting in the way of the healing they sincerely want to provide.

Engagement all flows from the leadership decisions we make. In fact, Gallup says that managers account for at least 70 percent of the variance in employee engagement across different areas of an organization.[18]

So what are the necessary conditions for each of these stakeholders—leaders, employees, clinicians, and patients—to engage? It turns out there are a number of evidence-based factors that are proven to increase engagement.

When it comes to leaders—senior leaders or even direct supervisors—their job is to create a work environment that encourages their employees (and physicians) to engage. Just as we can't force patients to engage, neither can we require employees or physicians to engage. We can, however, create a work environment that facilitates it. That's the role of the leader.

For example, by staying focused on the organization's mission, vision, and values, senior leaders can foster the kind of culture that is ripe for engagement. And I'm not talking about posting those words on the walls. I mean making sure they're walking through the halls, by role modeling and coaching the behaviors espoused in those documents. Furthermore, by ensuring appropriate compensation and benefits design, they ensure the organization can attract and retain a skilled workforce. Reward and recognition matters.

Direct supervisors also have unique duties. The truth is, they may even have a bigger impact on engagement than the senior leaders do. Communication is the key here. That includes setting clear expectations, both to start the year and for specific projects. And, they must provide clear and consistent feedback on progress to meeting those goals.

Feedback needs to be both transparent and timely, with an emphasis on the project itself and the person's development so he can maximize his potential.

For employees to be engaged, they must feel a sense of purpose, that their work is worthwhile and makes a difference. It's what drives all of us in healthcare. Also, their basic needs must be met. Gallup has identified that clear expectations are critical, and those expectations must be more than just a job description: "It's a detailed understanding of how what one person is supposed to do fits in with what everyone else is supposed to do and how those expectations change when circumstances change."[19] Employees want to feel valued and involved.

They also want a relationship with their supervisor. Studer Group recommends balancing compliments to criticism in a minimum of a three-to-one ratio to create a culture of positivity and a personal connection.

Gallup also says that employees are more likely to be engaged at work when they know what is expected and they have the materials and equipment to do their jobs.[20] As Gallup says, great managers are often the secret to unlocking the potential of high-performing employees. That holds true for engagement as well.

There are five things that drive physician engagement. The first is quality. Physicians want to know their patients are receiving quality care and a great patient experience. They also want to reduce the time it takes to follow up and address patient and family complaints.

The second is efficiency. Physicians want to work with team members who have the information needed to discuss their patients at hand. Over the course of a day, this will save physicians 30 minutes or more. The third is input. Physicians want a seat at the table to provide input when decisions are being made that affect clinical outcomes.

The fourth is responsive communication. They want to be kept current on how administration has positioned the organization to manage changes in the external environment and updated on things that will impact their patients or their practice.

And the final is appreciation. Physicians value a "thank-you" and acknowledgment when things are going well. They also want to see follow-through on their input in the form of tangible actions.

Engaged patients are activated patients. They trust their caregivers because they feel respected, understood, and cared about. They not only possess the information, skills, and confidence to actively participate in their care, but they also use it proactively to take action. They take ownership for their health through goal-setting.

Another important thing to understand: Engagement flows *down* from leaders to physicians/employees to patients and also flows *up* from patients to physicians/employees and leaders. It makes intuitive sense, doesn't it? If we're motivated in healthcare by a sense of purpose, worthwhile work, and making a difference, wouldn't we feel more engaged when individuals validate that for us?

> **Engagement flows *down* from leaders to physicians/ employees to patients and also flows *up* from patients to physicians/employees and leaders.**

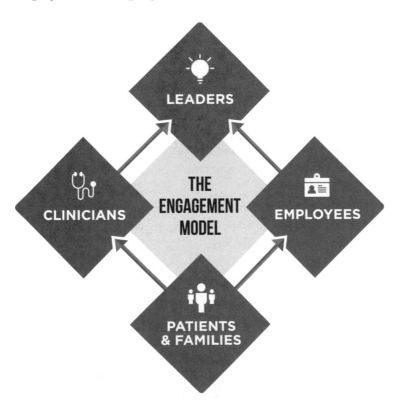

Figure 2.4 | Engagement also flows up, from patients to clinicians and employees and ultimately to leaders.

When a supervisor hears a thank-you from his employee for taking a personal interest in her professional development or useful feedback, he reengages. When an overweight patient shares with his physician that he's more engaged in his daily life because he lost weight and brought his blood pressure down thanks to his physician's intervention, that doctor is newly energized. He is reminded that he is doing sacred work healing patients and recommits to the rest of the patients he will see that day.

Hopefully by now, you're getting a sense of what a comprehensive strategy for engagement looks like. This brings me to an important point...

Putting Up a Portal Is Not an Engagement Strategy

We've already talked about how only engaged patients use patient portals anyway. At a minimum, we risk failing to reach our least engaged patients if this is all we do.

But the fact remains that if you Google "patient engagement" today, you're going to mostly read about technology, apps, and portals. These do play an important role in supporting effective patient engagement, and we will examine them further. In other words, they are necessary but insufficient.

Why are so many healthcare organizations rushing to put up portals? Financial incentives driven by federal meaningful use regulations for electronic health records, in large part. In 2015, the criteria for Stage 2 of meaningful use really raised the visibility of engagement.

These recommendations include three measures of engagement and require providers to successfully meet thresholds for two. Essentially, the government requires a percentage of a provider's patients—5 percent of them in 2015—to view, download, and transmit health data electronically, receive secure measures online, and contribute to patient-generated data.

And the stakes are high. In 2015, medical practices could earn up to $44,000 per physician over a five-year period from Medicare or up to $63,750 over six years from Medicaid by meeting these thresholds.[21] The problem is this has created a focus on getting the technology working quickly to optimize reimbursement.

With the rush to compliance, we've made a potentially dangerous detour by defining engagement too narrowly. Engagement is certainly much more than "connected health" online. And sometimes organizations, in their rush to check off their compliance with these regulations, don't even make much of an effort to make them patient-centered.

> **With the rush to compliance, we've made a potentially dangerous detour by defining engagement too narrowly. Engagement is certainly much more than "connected health" online.**

Recently, I switched to a new primary care physician myself and was delighted when the receptionist handed me a leaflet explaining that, after my first visit, I could access my information on their portal. But the login experience was cumbersome.

Once I finally got in, there was no information there. So I thought perhaps it would just take a few days to populate. But when I checked back a week later, there was still nothing there from my visit.

A few weeks later, I finally received an alert that said information had been added to my medical history so I went looking for my recent labs. But no, the only information available was a flu shot I'd received two years ago. I'm sure that particular portal is a fine portal, but for me, as a patient, it's not very useful. Certainly it did nothing to help engage me.

When it comes to engagement, what matters the most by far is human-to-human connection. That's what will truly make the difference, especially as technology continues to advance.

When I think back to the story I shared with you about my father-in-law's care, that's what mattered most to my wife. While I'm sure that Highlands

Rehabilitation Hospital has great technology behind the scenes, it's not what came to mind when I asked her to share what helped her and her family engage with their care.

It was the fact that Dr. Spier included her in the consultation on that pivotal afternoon. It was how caregivers sat with her and the key words they used at the bedside to calm and engage her dad. It's all about the *people*.

Key Learning Points: Engagement Is a Comprehensive Strategy

1. Engagement is a core organizational competency. Think of yourself as in the relationship business first and foremost.

2. Engagement is a higher order than satisfaction. Satisfaction is necessary but insufficient.

3. Patient Activation Measure—or PAM—represents an early effort to quantify and sort patients' engagement levels. Two key findings so far in research tracking PAM are that engaged patients have both lower costs and better outcomes.

4. Engagement starts with engaged leaders who create environments where clinicians can engage, who in turn facilitate patients' becoming engaged. And it works in reverse, too. It's a virtuous cycle of engagement.

5. Putting up a patient portal is not an engagement strategy. While it may be valuable for compliance with meaningful use regulations—and even for patients if it's well executed—we risk defining engagement far too narrowly if we consider it to just be "connected health" online.

PART TWO

What We Can Learn from Other Industries

Years ago, on the first day of one of my healthcare economics classes in graduate school, I watched the professor write the key rules of economics up on the blackboard and then cross them off one by one. So many of them, he said, don't apply to healthcare. The lack of price transparency, for example, means that basic principles of classical economics require adaptation when it comes to our industry.

More recently, I bumped into that very professor at a reception and told him how that lesson had remained vivid in my mind all these years later. "You know," he responded. "I'm scratching fewer and fewer principles off the board every year."

It was such a stark reminder to me that we really are feeling the effects in healthcare today of the true economic drivers of consumer behaviors. As consumers absorb an increasing share of the cost burden, they comparison shop. They're not hesitant at all to call up a hospital and ask about the cost of the procedure. In the same way, transparency with quality reporting—and even online patient experience reviews—means it's easy to see which hospital is safer or which doctor has a short wait and a great bedside manner.

Just think about the deluge of television and magazine advertising for prescription drugs. Consumers are responding by asking their doctors about these products. You can even find hospital ratings in *Consumer Reports* today.

In short, consumers are shopping for healthcare these days just like they've shopped for every other product in their lives. It may be alarming to us in healthcare, but it's the natural order of things. Clearly, it's time for healthcare to think like other industries do when it comes to building customer loyalty in all the ways that matter most. Not only will that be key to financial viability, but customer engagement strategies can also improve health outcomes.

CHAPTER 3

Lessons for Healthcare

As we've established, healthcare is undergoing tumultuous change. It's a disrupted industry. And what frequently happens in disrupted industries is a failure to fully appreciate the nature, extent, and velocity of the transformation that's occurring.

While the pace of change is challenging for those of us who work in healthcare, that's exactly what consultants and technology companies look for when scouting new opportunities: a market with great demand and the demographics to fuel growth in a business environment so disrupted by regulatory or pricing changes—or a need for innovation—that it's ripe for a new way of doing things.

In fact, they smell opportunity for new market entrants even as we struggle inside the industry with how to adapt to the twin pressures of higher quality and lower prices. The reality is that it's easier to build a new model than retrofit the old one. And agile companies—those that don't necessarily know much about healthcare but do have customer engagement as a core competency—are moving in.

Access Is King

What do customers want when it comes to healthcare? In large part, they want convenience and easy access. They want you to be open when they need you and located close by. Frankly, that's the major advantage that Walmart,

CVS, and other retailers enjoy as they move into medicine. They have an access advantage.

One of my colleagues at Huron Healthcare, Managing Director Ted Schwab, shared with me his experience a decade ago, when he helped a grocery store chain open a series of in-store clinics, well before companies like Walmart and CVS were doing it. He said the initial idea was to create easy access for less affluent customers who didn't have health insurance, so they made the service available on a cash-only basis.

To his surprise, the customers the clinics attracted were affluent. In fact, they were willing to pay a premium for the convenience of avoiding the complexity involved in scheduling and making it to an appointment in a doctor's office. When he surveyed patients about what was most important to them about their healthcare experience, they overwhelming responded that they cared most about convenience.

Think about it: If you call your doctor because you suspect you might have the flu, you'll be lucky if you can get a same-day appointment. And if you can, you'll probably need to leave work early or get pizza for the kids so you can get to the clinic at the dinner hour, if you're fortunate enough to have a doctor who offers evening appointments.

What if you think you might have strep throat on Saturday night? Imagine that you have a flight for an important business meeting on Monday. You need your throat looked at pronto. You *could* drive 20 minutes to the ER where you will pay a $1,000 deductible and will likely wait several hours to be seen by a doctor.

Or, in either of these two scenarios above, you could just swing by the CVS MinuteClinic in your neighborhood when it's convenient. The clinics are open seven days a week (holidays and weekends included), no appointment necessary. You likely won't even wait. Plus, they accept most insurance plans, and it might cost you $40 to $60 total. If you do need a prescription, you're already conveniently at the pharmacy to fill it.

According to a survey by the Advisory Board Company, patients said they would rather get seen without an appointment and have access to night and weekend hours than see an actual physician.[1] When asked about their top 10 preferred attributes of a primary care clinic, the number-one attribute was "I can walk in without an appointment, and I'm guaranteed to be seen within 30 minutes."[2] Maybe that's why it's so easy to log onto CVS online, view the actual wait time at your local clinic, and click the "hold place in line" button—if there is a wait—while you drive over.

Walgreens, CVS, and Walmart aren't pursuing the 40 percent of potential patients who already have a primary care physician and are comfortable dealing with the complexity of healthcare. They're pursuing the other 60 percent. It turns out that between 40 and 50 percent of their patients have no regular primary care provider.[3]

They are pursuing the working mom who is already stopping by the pharmacy who wants to get that cough checked out if she finds herself with an extra 10 minutes…and the millennial who isn't interested in decoding the healthcare industry when she needs contraceptive care…and the business executive who needs a quick sports physical so he can turn in that form for the softball league at work.

Retail clinics are growing quickly in response to demand. In fact, the number of clinics has increased sevenfold in the past eight years, to a total of 1,866 nationwide in 2015.[4] It's predicted that globally, the number of patients who visit them will jump from 15.1 million in 2015 to 30.7 million in 2022.[5] CVS is the market leader with close to 1,000 locations and 18 million patient visits in 2013.[6]

And one trend that's driving that demand is the physician shortage. In fact, the Association of American Medical Colleges predicts that by 2025, the U.S. faces a shortfall of up to 94,700 physicians, including up to 35,600 primary care physicians.[7] But it's easy to see a nurse practitioner or physician assistant at a retail clinic. The most common conditions patients seek treatment for at these retail clinics are respiratory, sinus, ear, throat, eye, and urinary tract infections, as well as immunizations.[8]

So are retail clinics a new best practice that represents the future of health-care? A great replacement for primary care? Most definitely not. Yet, we can't dismiss them out of hand as "bad medicine." To the contrary, several studies show they are delivering care on par or superior to conventional options. We ignore this trend at our own peril.

Instead, let's look at what they're doing right and understand what we can learn as an industry from the way they put patients at the center of care. The reality is that healthcare consumers today are voting with both their feet and their wallets, and we ignore their choices at our own risk.

Influencing Consumer Behavior Is Key to Engagement

While it's true that the clinics enjoy a big advantage in customer engagement due to their convenient hours and locations, that's really only part of the se-cret sauce that differentiates them. One of their unique competencies—one that we haven't focused on yet in healthcare—is their ability to influence consumer behavior.

It would probably come as no surprise to you that retailers you shop with are tracking your data today. Right now, they may use what they know about your past purchasing patterns to encourage you to buy a related product. That's how Netflix knows which next movie you might like and Amazon knows which products to recommend. In the future, though, they will be able to crunch that data to predict what you'll buy and use it to their advantage. In fact, you might be surprised that they know what you need before you do.

Target already excels at this. In fact, a few years ago, after analyzing its shop-pers' buying habits, it decided to take aim at pregnant women as a rich source of consumers about to purchase lots of baby items.[9] (It turns out that new shopping habits—like all habits—are incredibly hard to shape and reset ex-cept during key life events like getting married and having a baby.)

By analyzing purchases, Target determined that if it could capture women in their second trimester of pregnancy, it could likely beat out potential compet-itors who would ply them with discounts and coupons after the baby was born and retain them as customers for years.

So analysts went to work to determine which shoppers were pregnant. Since Target assigns each shopper a Guest ID that tracks what each person buys and links it to all kinds of demographic information, it was easy to overlay data the company buys about ethnicity, job history, college, home ownership, and more.

Statisticians determined that women on Target's baby registry bought more unscented lotion and supplements, among other items, in their second trimester, which then allowed them to assign a "pregnancy predictor score" and estimate a due date to send coupons timed to specific stages of the pregnancy.

Unfortunately, in one instance, a very angry father showed up at a store to speak with a manager when Target started sending diaper coupons to his teenage daughter. He worried they were promoting promiscuity, but later apologized when he learned she actually *was* pregnant and hadn't shared the news with him yet.

(I had a similar experience myself, actually. Right when I was immersed in learning about Target's genius approach to targeting future customers, I opened my mailbox at home one day to find a coupon for diapers addressed to my wife! We did not have any children in diapers. Fortunately, when I showed her the postcard and asked her if there was anything she wanted to share with me, she said she'd been planning a baby shower for our babysitter.)

Target has since worked to avoid such public relations nightmares by refining its marketing to be more circumspect. Now, instead of sending overt postcards for a host of pacifiers, sanitizers, and diapers in the mail, pregnant women find those offers mixed into flyers that also pointedly include sales on lawnmowers and other innocuous items to avoid offense.

Each flyer is completely customized for the intended recipient, although she would never guess that's the case. (If you squint, you can almost imagine a time in the future when your cell phone approaches Target's front doors to relay data that automatically assembles a welcome basket of goods custom-selected for you. Can you see it?)

How will you compete with the likes of Target and CVS when it comes to healthcare? There's a vast scientific basis behind all of this data crunching, combining predictive analytics with behavioral economics and other disciplines to influence consumer behavior. Today, that's being used to induce repeat purchases, loyalty to the brand, bigger purchases, and more. But what if that same know-how could be applied to influence healthcare behaviors?

Some of these new entrants into the healthcare market are bringing this use of big data to predict future behaviors that actually influence consumer behavior. They're studying the neuroscience of how to break bad habits and create positive ones and apply it to tough challenges like chronic diseases... to influence whether a particular patient actually takes that medicine as prescribed and takes charge of her own health.

Walgreens clinics, for instance, will diagnose and treat conditions like asthma, diabetes, and high blood pressure.[10] It's a bold move and a potentially lucrative one too, as those patients represent repeat customers for Walgreens' medical supplies and prescription drugs.

As an industry, we can either learn from those organizations on the frontiers of harnessing customer information or ignore their success at our own peril. One of the things CVS is currently tackling with digital technology is the epidemic of people who don't stay on their medication schedule. CVS actually sends text reminders to 20 million customers so they don't forget.[11]

Plans are underway at CVS to take this approach to the next level by adding a capability for prescription reminders into the CVS mobile app...even allowing customers to enter a friend's name who can be alerted if they miss a dose. Also in development at CVS: connecting third-party medical devices to smartphones to take a video of a patient's ear and then send it to Minute-Clinic pharmacists for instant diagnosis and subsequent prescription for ear infections.[12]

Target won't be left out of this one-stop shopping approach to healthcare either. In fact, it's already launched clinics in seven states, offering more than

60 services, with the capacity to see up to 60 patients per day. It's even teamed up with Kaiser Permanente to staff several clinics in southern California.[13]

Think about the power of this retail model for a moment in terms of follow-up visits. I suspect that patients are less likely to cancel those appointments when they need to swing by Target next week anyway to stock up on toilet paper and juice boxes.

Uber will see you now. If it's not enough that retailers are moving into the healthcare space, there's Uber. Far from posing as just another taxicab service, Uber is quick to identify gaps between demand and supply of services and then capitalize on them. In fact, Uber *specializes* in matching unmet demand with unused supply...in all kinds of things.

The company began, of course, by pairing ride seekers who didn't want the hassle, high fares, or awkward tipping experience of cabs with car owners who could use a little extra cash. But from there, they've expanded into a number of interesting ventures. For one thing, Uber offers Christmas tree deliveries on demand in November and December.

If you live in a sixth floor apartment in Manhattan and detest lugging a Christmas tree up all those steps, you'll be delighted to know that you can select "CHRISTMAS TREE" in the Uber app and enjoy a direct delivery. No fumbling for your credit card either. Uber takes the $110 fee automatically from your credit card on file.

In October 2015, Uber even paired up with an animal shelter to offer kittens for cuddling. Here's how it worked: If you opened the Uber app on the specified day between 11 a.m. and 3 p.m. and requested "KITTENS," they'd be delivered for the best 15 minutes of your day for just a $30 snuggle fee. A bonus: In most cities, kittens are eligible for adoption.

Uber even offers on-demand flu shots in winter.[14] It all started back in the winter of 2014, when John Brownstein, an epidemiologist at Boston Children's Hospital and Harvard Medical School, wondered about a better way to get around the problem of low vaccination rates (only 30 percent of adults get them, according to the Centers for Disease Control and Prevention).

When speaking with potential patients, people said they weren't opposed to the shots. Rather, they skipped them because it was inconvenient to make a doctor's appointment since it wasn't part of their usual routine. As a result, Brownstein worked with Uber to offer a medical professional in an Uber car to deliver shots for $10.

Since that individual can give up to 10 flu shots at each location for no extra charge, it's easy to split the cost with coworkers, too. The one-day effort was so successful—with more than 2,000 vaccinations in Boston, New York, Washington, and Chicago—that Uber and its partners scaled up in winter of 2015 to reach individuals in 35 cities nationwide. When Brownstein and researchers surveyed those who used Uber to get the shots in 2104, nearly 80 percent said they wouldn't have had the vaccine if it weren't for Uber.[15]

From a public health standpoint, this is a good thing. Even those of us who didn't get the flu shot benefit directly from others' immunity. It's good medicine because it closed the gap for those who weren't opposed to the vaccine, but weren't likely to get it otherwise.

Is this the direction healthcare is heading? It's clearly not the answer to closing the gap in economic disparities within healthcare. It's a convenient service for those who have the cash to pay for it.

However, it's an example of a novel and high-impact approach to meeting patient needs by one company that doesn't think of its core competency as healthcare delivery. They're focused instead on consumer engagement. This is the power of engagement at work.

Are We *Consumers* or *Patients*?

Remember the story I shared about my professor crossing off all the ways the healthcare industry didn't comply with basic rules of economics?

The other thing I remember from that first day of class is how the professor used the term *consumer* rather than *patient*. One of my classmates—a physician, actually—took exception to that word. He explained that "in medicine, we prefer the word 'patient.'"

The professor's response? He said that sometimes the difference between a consumer and a patient is simply how vertical you are at a given moment. In other words, if you're walking around and have a choice, you're a consumer. If you're lying on an operating table, you're a patient.

Consider having this discussion with the team at your organization. Ask them what they see as the key differences between patients and consumers and which strategies you use to account for their different needs. In your system, hospital, or medical practice, do you organize around *patients*...or do you organize around *consumers*? If we're honest, the likely answer will be neither. Typically, we organize around our own needs as practitioners. And that's a problem.

> **In your system, hospital, or medical practice, do you organize around *patients*...or do you organize around *consumers*?**

It's important to bring awareness to this tendency...and to the fact that everyone on your team may perceive the patient's role differently. I had a particularly illuminating experience with respect to this at a strategic planning retreat I facilitated for Columbia Valley Community Health (CVCH), a federally qualified healthcare organization in Wenatchee, WA, several years ago.

At the retreat, the CEO of CVCH, Patrick Bucknum, broke his team of 15 leaders into five groups of three and gave them each a flip chart. Next, he asked them to go to the corners of the room with the flip charts facing toward the wall so no one could see what anyone else was writing. He next asked them to draw the key players in a football game and then to label each of them as if they were the various stakeholders at Columbia Valley.

In other words, which player would be the patient? The doctor? The nurses? Which one would be the healthcare administrators? Or the regulators? Or the payers? As I walked around the room, I was surprised how differently each team saw them. One group saw the patient as the quarterback while another group saw the patient as the ball. Another group saw the patient as a spectator, while another one saw them as the referee.

Bucknum then turned all the flipcharts around so we could examine the differences. He talked about what it means if you perceive the patient as the ball versus the quarterback or the spectator. How would we organize ourselves differently if we each shared the same vision of the patient at the center of care?

And to put this exercise in context, CVCH and its leaders are among the very best I've worked with at putting the patient at the center of what they do. As with all federally qualified health centers, they are far more patient-centric than most other types of providers.

It starts with their governance structure, which requires a minimum 51 percent composition from patients they serve, and it extends into the physical design of the clinics, the training of staff, and the metrics they track for improvement. And yet even here at CVCH, at one of the very best, there's a wide diversity of perspectives about the role the patient plays on the team.

In his book *Being Mortal*, Atul Gawande touches on this very challenge in nursing homes today. He explains that the nursing home experience is completely designed around efficiencies that benefit the staff rather than the patient.[16]

Think about it: Patients must wake up at a certain time so the staff can bathe and feed them when it's convenient for the staff to deliver the therapies and treatments they need. Patients take medications on a schedule that is convenient for the pharmacist. It's not that we're self-centered and callous to the needs of our patients. As Dr. Gawande points out, what we want for others is *safety*; what we want for ourselves is *autonomy*.

If, instead, we organized around the needs of the patients, they'd wake up when they felt like it and go to breakfast when they were hungry. Wouldn't that give us a sense of control later in life as nursing home patients? Perhaps we wouldn't dread our stay there quite so much.

Of course, from an operator's standpoint, it seems impossible to redesign the system around residents. And yet, that's exactly what new treatment facilities are doing. Increasingly, independent living concepts are emerging where you can enjoy as much autonomy as you like, as long as you're willing to accept the accompanying risks.

Try This Exercise: Kill the Company

Imagine this scenario with your team: You are your organization's main competitor with unlimited resources. Or a new market entrant with roots in technology or retail. What would you do to your organization right now to put it out of business?

In her book *Kill the Company*, author Lisa Bodell challenges readers to cut to the chase in their quest for innovation by using this exercise.[17] Sure, you could use a SWOT analysis to examine strengths, weaknesses, opportunities, and threats, but if you really want to understand where the big problems and opportunities lie when it comes to creating a culture of engagement, try this instead: Ask your team what they'd do to kill the company.

Then prioritize threats and consider solutions. (See Lisa's book for complete details.) The typical answer on how to kill the company? You'd completely reinvent the healthcare delivery organization from a patient-centered perspective.

Instead of asking your patients to wander through a maze of buildings for an in-person appointment with a doctor and wait 30 minutes or more, maybe you'd let them access an app from home when it worked for them. In short, you'd make things easy, convenient, and efficient because that's what people value.

And that's exactly what new competitors who excel at engagement are doing today. Get ready.

Are You a Fox or a Hedgehog?

There is an ancient Greek parable by philosopher Archilochus that distinguishes between a fox, which knows many things, and a hedgehog, which knows one important thing. In Jim Collins's seminal book, *Good to Great*, he points out that all great leaders are hedgehogs. They know how to simplify a complex world into a single, organizing idea—the kind of basic principle that unifies, organizes, and guides all decisions.

That's not to say that hedgehogs are simplistic. They're like great thinkers, who take complexities and boil them down into simple, yet profound, ideas. (Think of Adam Smith and the invisible hand...or Darwin and evolution.)

This is true for companies, too. The likes of Target, CVS, and Uber are all hedgehogs. They understand customer engagement first and foremost and they know how to apply it in new ventures. To learn from their example—and construct our own hedgehog concept—we need to ask three pivotal questions. First, what can we be best in the world at? (And equally important, what can we *not* be best at?)

Second, what is the economic denominator that best drives our economic engine (i.e., our profit or cash flow per unit)? And finally, what are our core people deeply passionate about?

Warren Buffett calls that a moat of competitive advantage that separates you and your organization from competitors. As a rule, Buffett invests only in businesses that are castles with moats. He describes them as wonderful businesses with durable competitive advantages. Castle-and-moat businesses are built upon a winning business strategy and strategic brand that have high barriers to competitor imitation and entry.

What distinguishes your organization in this way? How wide is *your* moat? And what is it filled with? I believe that to survive and thrive today and far into the future, the answer must be customer engagement.

Key Learning Points: Lessons for Healthcare

1. Access is king. CVS MinuteClinic, Walmart, and Target are mushrooming because consumers value convenience even higher than seeing a doctor.

2. Influencing consumer behavior is key to engagement. Predictive analytics and real-time patient data can likely increase a patient's commitment to following a care plan, improve clinical quality, reduce no-shows, and more.

3. Marketing entrants into healthcare are capitalizing on matching unmet demand with unused supply.

4. Healthcare organizations must find a way to put patients at the center of their care. When we design systems and processes around our own convenience instead of theirs, we create a critical misalignment with what's most important to patients, leading to disengagement.

PART THREE

How to Engage Stakeholders Critical to Our Success

The wonderful thing about engagement is that the principle is the same... whether we're talking about leaders, employees, clinicians, or even patients. People who feel valued—as well as a sense of trust, responsibility, and empowerment—are just more likely to engage.

The best way to inspire engagement is to connect with both our hearts and our minds. Authenticity, for example, is a vital component of connecting with another human being. It builds the trust that's necessary to create a culture of engagement, which is a precursor to high performance.

Empathy is another important ingredient in inspiring trust from another human being. When we have empathy, people trust us. They know we care about them. Every data point I've ever read says that when someone feels cared about as a person, they listen better and are more comfortable asking questions and asking for help. Like the old adage says, "No one cares how much you know until they know how much you care."

One of the most effective ways to show empathy as a leader is the willingness to show vulnerability. Don't be afraid to share your own successes, struggles, and mistakes. Remember, no one goes through life undefeated. When leaders stand with employees through personal victories and challenges, they become more likely to engage in the organization that supports them. Employees take notice of values-driven leaders, those who make decisions aligned with the organization's values. They feel good about working with leaders who create consistency in the workplace.

Empathy means approaching other people with the full awareness and disclosure that we too are human and have flaws. But we never quit trying to get better and better. It's the same with caregivers who show empathy to patients. Patients feel and respond to their willingness to connect.

Perhaps the most important way we encourage engagement is to connect the dots for people in a way that creates clear understanding and leads to the outcomes we're seeking. Make sure the listener understands the desired outcome first. Then explain how to do it, and, if you can, share a story that illustrates the impact. It works with leaders, employees, clinicians, and patients.

Sure, some people are naturals when it comes to authenticity, demonstrating empathy, and communicating clearly, but you know what? Even those of us who tend to be a little more reserved or a little less articulate can also become adept at these skills with practice.

The vast majority of us already use both our minds and our hearts to make decisions and take action. With a little willingness to build our skills and commit to better connecting with others at work, we can connect even more powerfully to create and sustain a culture of high engagement.[1]

CHAPTER 4

Engaging Employees (A Requisite for Leaders)

If engagement is the answer to transforming healthcare—delivering higher quality to patients at a lower cost—how do our employees factor into the equation? The truth is it's two sides of the same coin. Engaged employees allow us to realize both of these aims, while disengaged employees cause us to miss both marks. Let's look at quality first.

One of the most frustrating patient safety issues in healthcare today is the challenge of consistent hand hygiene. The reason it's so frustrating is that it's very clear that people know they should wash their hands to reduce infections, and they know how to do it, but all too often they just don't do it. It's the ultimate "knowing-doing" gap.

Early on, leaders scratched their heads and worked hard to eliminate any barriers to hand hygiene that they could think of. Do we have enough sinks in the right places? Are the foam dispensers filled? Are the schedules packed so tightly that clinicians can't find five seconds to wash their hands? But none of these things closed the gap.

And that's a serious problem. The Centers for Disease Control and Prevention estimates there are 1.7 million hospital-acquired infections annually, leading to 99,000 deaths in the U.S.[1] The fact is, the most common way to transmit pathogens is via hands. So this lack of handwashing is the biggest source of hospital-acquired infections.[2, 3]

Despite the fact that consistent handwashing is our best defense against in-fections, the national average for handwashing is about 50 percent.[4] But here's the really interesting thing: One study showed that there is a near-perfect correlation between handwashing compliance and employee engagement.[5] It showed conclusively that as engagement increases, so does handwashing.

This is perhaps not surprising. If engagement is really about what the em-ployee is doing when nobody is watching, then hand hygiene is a great quality marker of an engaged employee. In the end, what will most improve compli-ance with hand hygiene protocol is clinicians who choose to do it every time because it's the right thing to do for patients. Really, it's about commitment, not just compliance.

Engaged Employees Do It Right

Early in my career, my focus was on quality and safety. I had a mentor during those years who shared with me a story that really illustrates the impact of disengaged employees on quality. She worked with an organization that had revised their policy to eliminate restraints.

While some believe there are times that patients need to be physically re-strained for safe care—in the midst of a psychotic episode or seizure instance, for example—most organizations have long since moved away from the use of the kinds of belts and straps that used to be used, with rare exceptions. Today, we understand there are better options in restraint-free environments that can avoid some of the dangers of those old-fashioned restraints.

In any case, after revising the policy, leaders at this particular organization pulled all the restraints out of inventory and trained everyone on the new way of doing things. You couldn't even order the restraints anymore. Imagine her surprise then, when they had a restraint-related death six months later.

Upon investigation, they found there had been a work around. Certain em-ployees had hoarded the old restraints and continued to use them. Why? Busy, well-intentioned professionals will work around systems they don't be-lieve have value. It's not that they're bad people or that they're trying to harm patients; rather, they haven't internalized the value proposition of doing the behavior in the new way. That's what engaged employees do.

Dr. Grant Savage, a professor at the Collat School of Business at the University of Alabama at Birmingham, has studied this phenomenon specifically and found that employees who are not very engaged are dramatically more likely to use work-around safety procedures than highly engaged employees.

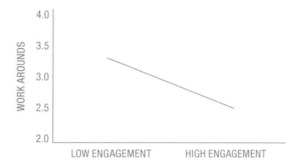

Figure 4.1 | Employees who are less engaged are more likely to work around safety protocols.

Source: Leroy, Hannes et al. "Behavioral Integrity for Safety, Priority of Safety, Psychological Safety, and Patient Safety: A Team-Level Study." *Journal of Applied Psychology* 97 no.6 (2012): 1273-1281. doi:10.1037/a0030076.

I also remember my excitement when barcode administration of medications first rolled out back in the late '90s. As someone who was spending a lot of my time working with organizations to reduce medication errors, the new technology seemed so promising.

After all, if you have to scan the medication, scan the patient's ID, and can give the medication only when there is a match, how could you ever again deliver a medication to the wrong patient? And yet, it turns out that busy professionals who haven't embraced the value of the new approach will find a work around.

In this case, I remember my disappointment upon reading cases where care-givers defeated the system by simply printing off additional patient ID bar codes at the nursing station. They scanned all of the meds and all of the patient IDs at one convenient time and then walked around to distribute them, instead of scanning the ID actually on the patient's wrist as was expected.

This is the same phenomenon we've frequently seen with surgery time outs. The concept, of course, is that before the team performs a procedure, they huddle, review the facts of the case, and confirm the specific body part that will be operated on to avoid an error. If anyone disagrees, they speak up and say so.

My colleague, Davy Crockett (yes, that's really his name…he's a descendant of the legend!), a coach at Studer Group®, has shared with me that he's seen great variability by pre-operative unit with respect to this practice depending on the level of their engagement. The challenge, of course, is that 99.9 percent of the time these huddles are routine and don't overtly intercept an error.

It could be tempting to skip it and consider it a waste of time. However, a highly engaged team understands that consistent practice of the huddle is necessary to catch a potential error for the .1 percent of the time those errors actually occur.

You know who understands the importance of following safety checklists? Pilots. My brother is a pilot with Delta Airlines. He's a great example of someone who identified his career passion at a young age. I remember when he was around nine and I was six, my dad bought a new washing machine. Chris dragged the box upstairs and a few hours later he'd turned it into a cockpit of an A-10 attack aircraft.

At 12, he started building and flying remote-controlled planes. And then at 15, he started flying the real thing. We didn't realize at the time how unusual it was that he could take me up in a plane and fly a few states over, but he couldn't drive me home since he received his pilot's license before his driver's license! (Mom would have to come pick us up in the minivan.)

Chris received a degree in aviation and then at 21 began flying with a commercial airline. It's a profession he's had now for more than 20 years, but a passion he's had for twice as long.

Like me, Chris is interested in safety. And we've often discussed the differences between aviation and medicine. For example, just as we use checklists in surgery, so do pilots use checklists before a flight. But while the compliance with checklists in surgery is highly variable, the adoption of aviation checklists is very high.

It's cultural. My brother Chris would never consider skipping the checklist for his jet, even though he's flown over 10,000 hours. Going through the checklist isn't considered an affront to his professionalism or intelligence. In fact, the whole point of the checklist is to offload the basic tasks that are routine to reserve vigilance and focus for the higher order tasks that require expertise. It's truly a job aid.

High Employee Engagement Reduces Turnover

One of the fastest growing segments of our business at Studer Group is coaching the leaders of organizations who ask us to support their employee engagement initiatives because they want to reduce employee turnover. Today, we're seeing organizations that used to have turnover in the single digits now watching it rise to above 20 percent.

That kind of turnover represents a tremendous financial cost to the organization. If the average cost of replacing an employee is $60,000 or more (when you include recruitment, vacancy, transition, and orientation costs), just think about the expense of high turnover. An organization losing 20 percent of its 3,000 employees with an average salary of $45,000 is racking up costs of $27 million per year. Just a 1 percent reduction in turnover means an additional $1.3 million returned to the organization.[6] What could you do with an extra $1.3 million?

But even more important than their desire to dramatically reduce turnover, we find that organizations increasingly are asking for our help in improving employee engagement because they understand that they can't transform healthcare without it.

Healthcare organizations are not just being asked to do things better than we have in the past; we're being asked to do things differently. If we're going to reinvent the healthcare industry to compete with the Ubers and CVSs of the world, as we discussed in Chapter 3, we'll need every one of our people to bring their creativity, commitment, and best ideas to succeed.

> **Healthcare organizations are not just being asked to do things better than we have in the past; we're being asked to do things differently.**

Think about it: It doesn't matter how good our technology is if nobody uses it...or how good the capital plan is if we fail in the execution. As our need to transform healthcare becomes more urgent, so does the need to really hone in on the people side of change.

At Studer Group, we know that if you engage your people around your mission and your strategy, the rest really falls into place. We see it happen every day in thousands of health systems, community hospitals, and physician organizations that we coach across North America and Australia.

Values and Passion Drive Employee Engagement

This notion of engaging employees is at the very foundation of our belief system at Studer Group. Our mission is to create better places for *employees to work*, physicians to practice medicine, and patients to receive care. And our vision talks about maximizing the *human potential* within our healthcare industry. If there's one thing that's true, it's that sustainably excellent organizations have strong people engagement systems.

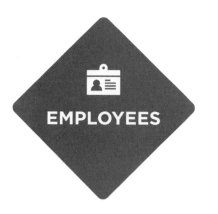

What drives employee engagement?

• Purposeful, worthwhile work

• Feeling valued and involved

• Relationship with supervisor

• Opportunities

Figure 4.2 | Understand the drivers for employee engagement.

In fact, the model that guides our work is the Healthcare Flywheel®, which shows that the pathway to transforming and sustaining high-performing organizations starts with engaging the employees.

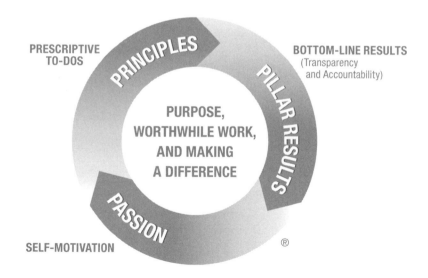

Figure 4.3 | The Healthcare Flywheel® turns when individuals feel that they have purposeful, worthwhile work that makes a difference.

If you can connect the dots between an evidence-based practice that employees ought to be doing and their commitment to having purposeful, meaningful work that makes a difference in the lives of others, they're likely to commit to doing that practice.

One of my favorite analogies is my boys' love of soccer. When Julie's dad was diagnosed with his brain tumor, we really focused on ensuring our boys learned about and spent time with him in those remaining months. They were fascinated with his years playing professional soccer.

I reminded them that they have *his* genes; they have that same potential. I loved watching how this lit a fire in them. While they'd enjoyed soccer in the years prior to when I made this connection for them, this put them over the top. If the weather is nice and they have some free time at home, you can find them in the backyard for hours at a time using the two small goals we set up for them. They found the passion.

But passion alone is insufficient. You have to have both *will* and *skill*. My sons are fortunate to also have great coaches at the YMCA where they play, who teach them the fundamentals. And when they apply those skills with passion, they see the results.

Yes, sometimes they score a goal and sometimes their team wins. But what I'm talking about here is the feeling of success that comes from knowing you did your best and produced good results: solid passes, nice defense, listening to the coach, staying in space instead of clumping up.

I can see it on their faces when they're playing and hear it as we debrief on the game going home. (Of course, as a Studer Group dad, I always ask them "what worked well" and "what could be even better next time.") And that feeling of success fires them up even more. It's how the flywheel spins: Find what you love, get good at it, and celebrate the results.

There's No Such Thing as *"Just a…"* in Healthcare

There's no such thing in healthcare as *just a* housekeeper or *just a* maintenance guy. My Studer Group colleague Rich Bluni often shares the story of his dad who worked as a maintenance foreman in a hospital up until he passed away.

He says he remembers once when he was just a kid hearing someone ask his dad what he did for a living and his dad replied, "I work in healthcare." Then the person asked, "Aren't you just a maintenance guy?"

The question took his dad aback for a moment because he didn't think of himself that way. But he didn't get mad. Instead he explained: "If I consider myself just a maintenance guy and I don't take what I do seriously every day, there can be serious consequences. Imagine if a generator went out during a big storm because I didn't think it was that important to test them regularly…because I'm *just a* maintenance guy.

"What if a team was in the OR at that moment in the middle of a life-saving surgery? If they are working in the dark and none of the equipment works, someone could die. So I never look at anything I do from the perspective of being just a…"

While a nurse's *job* may be documenting, his *work* is caring for patients and relieving pain. A housekeeper's *job* may be mopping floors and emptying trash, but his *work* is preventing infections to save people's lives. It's the *work* that inspires us.

So remember—the next time you hear yourself or someone else say, *"I'm just a…,"* redirect them. There's no such thing as *just a* in healthcare.

My colleague coach Barbara Hotko describes the Healthcare Flywheel as similar to how the flywheel on a steam engine drives a train.[7] She says, "When you listen to the sound of the engine, you can hear the push that starts the engine. Then as the engine moves, the train gains momentum, until the momentum is so great, it's difficult to stop. Some say it takes eight miles for a locomotive to stop."

It's the same with the Healthcare Flywheel. Employees' passion for doing important work fuels their willingness to use tools and tactics that get results. Results generate increasing momentum for more results on the journey to excellence until they are "hardwired." In other words, an organization can sustain the gains, even if great leaders come and go.

When we see organizations struggle to get results, it's rarely because they aren't familiar with best practices. Rather, it's that they haven't been able to sustainably execute those practices. Often, the difference between excellence and mediocrity is consistency.

> **Often, the difference between excellence and mediocrity is consistency.**

There's variation in who executes to the plan and how often. In time, if the positive behaviors are ignored, people engage in those behaviors less frequently. And if the negative behaviors are ignored, they increase. The result is that the performance improvement gains slide back down to the baseline, change then stalls, and the organization assumes the practice "just doesn't work here." What doesn't work there is their systematic approach for getting people to do the things that evidence suggests are the right things to do.

Evidence-Based Leadership Is Built for Employee Engagement

The pathway we advise organizations to follow to close this gap between knowing and doing is the same leadership operating system we use within Studer Group ourselves. Evidence-Based Leadership[SM] is an execution framework that uses aligned goals to create aligned behavior so that people apply aligned processes to hardwire sustainable results.

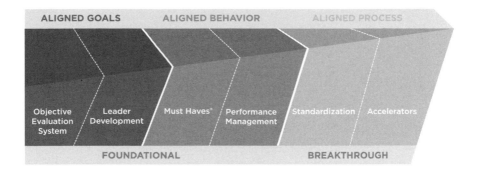

Figure 4.4 | Aligned goals foster aligned behavior to use aligned processes that hardwire results.

When most organizations contemplate how to make improvements, whether they want to improve a specific metric in a narrow area of the organization or address something larger and transformative, they often consider various process improvement modalities. One that's been particularly popular in healthcare is the Lean methodology that was adopted from the Toyota production model. We've learned a lot about this in recent months as we began working with the deep team of process improvement experts within Safer Healthcare, now part of Huron.

It's a smart approach. They begin by identifying the underlying processes and then work toward improving those, by eliminating the waste and reducing unwarranted variation in the design of the process. The result is an ideally designed process.

And that's essential to making meaningful improvement. However, that's just the beginning of the journey to achieve a sustainable outcome. Because next you need to ensure that people will actually perform that process in the optimal way…forever. And that's where traditional process improvement breaks down.

Years ago, I conducted an employee focus group with an internal process improvement group at a large, well-known academic medical center. They were incredibly frustrated. And I quickly understood why.

In the prior year, the director of their lab asked for help from this team to improve turnaround time for their lab specimens. So the process improvement (PI) team worked with the lab team to design a new, agile process. By all accounts, it was ideally designed. The lab began using the new process, and the PI team moved on to their next project.

Months later, however, the lab director called back to share his frustration that turnaround time of lab specimens was once again a challenge. The PI team met again with the team, only to find that the original process had crept back into place. The new process was nowhere to be seen. (Does this remind you of the work-around stories I shared earlier?)

Following Studer Group's Evidence-Based Leadership model, I asked them: "Who has accountability for the outcome of the process? In other words, who is responsible for, measured on, and evaluated on the success of turnaround time of lab specimens?" The answer: Nobody.

The lab director was evaluated on a subjective, narrative-based annual evaluation. The only metrics he was clearly accountable for related to the budget. So that meant that turnaround time was a "department goal" that was being reported out on some scorecard, although no individual had accountability. Maybe they used the old philosophy that "everyone in the department" was accountable for the goal. (Studer Group would counter that if everyone's accountable, then *no one's* accountable.)

The reality is: Culture eats process improvement for lunch. A culture of high engagement is facilitated first by setting clear accountability with transparent goals. Now, you didn't hear me say that process improvement isn't necessary. Of course, it's essential. But unless you have accountability for the outcome of that process, you'll allow barriers and excuses to get in the way of sustainable results.

A culture of high engagement is facilitated first by setting clear accountability with transparent goals.

Most organizations have solid accountability at the top. There is typically a robust balanced scorecard with red, yellow, and green highlighting progress or lack of progress toward the goal across a balanced set of measures.

Where this approach breaks down is that this accountability doesn't frequently cascade those measures (and that accountability) to the leaders who have the most influence over the results. And yet, Gallup research indicates that clear expectations are at the very bedrock of an engaged workplace.[8]

Getting data isn't usually the problem. Rather, making sense of it is. I often ask leaders to estimate how many things are counted at their organization. Is the answer a single digit number? Double digit? Triple digit?

I'd venture that most audiences I speak to work at places that track hundreds, if not thousands, of measures. So which of those are *key*? Each of them is likely important to someone and some function; the key is to divide and conquer.

The goal is to identify the handful of measures that give that leader the information they need to make the best decisions. Think about your car, for example. If you've purchased it in the past few years, it has a computer, capturing hundreds of metrics continuously. Each is important to some aspect of performance. But how many of those does it display to the driver at any one time to help you make decisions? Most likely, you see a handful of them… maybe three to five, to focus your attention on what matters most.

In the same way, Studer Group advises organizations to identify the six to eight key metrics that best reflect the aims of the organization. Then, cascade those goals so that each individual leader has their own, unique six to eight goals they can control or influence. The annual results on those metrics ought to comprise 100 percent of that individual's year-end evaluation.

But that's only a small part of what's required of a systematic accountability system that hardwires great results. In fact, knowing the results at the end of the year is like knowing the score of the baseball game for the first time once the game is over. How does that help the team win the game? Clearly, it doesn't.

What helps ensure you're making progress toward those key goals is a monthly conversation about year-to-date results on each metric, so you can adjust your action plans over the next 90 days as needed. This ensures that the supervisor and their direct report are aligned, that barriers are being identified, and that new short-term projects don't distract from critical long-term goals.

As Gallup explains, "Employees require more than a self-established job description; they want someone to talk with them regularly about their responsibilities and progress. Clarity of expectations is vital to performance."[9]

How does this relate to engagement? I can tell you from having used this system for the past 10 years within Studer Group that high performers love it. By their very nature, high performers are driven to exceed goals, problem solve, and bring solutions.

They are highly committed to making things better for their unit and the organization as a whole, so they love clarity around what's expected and frequent communication on how they can get there efficiently. In other words, they're highly engaged. So goal-setting and quarterly conversations are tools to re-recruit your best employees and avoid those turnover costs I shared earlier.

Leader development ensures your people know *how* to do what you're asking. There's an old adage that if people don't do the things that evidence suggests they ought to do, it's either because they don't want to (as we've established) or they don't know how to do it. Leader development is all about eliminating the possibility that they don't know how to do it.

While each organization will approach leadership development differently, there are some common elements we find in world-class organizations with respect to how they develop talents on the leadership team. First, if you're going to invest the significant resources that are required to elevate your leadership team, the first principle of training ought to be that attendance is mandatory, not optional.

Think about it: Who shows up to optional training? The very people who don't need it: your high performers, the individuals who are enlightened enough to know that professional development is valuable.

The second thing world-class organizations do is commit to a high frequency of training. Studer Group has found that it is helpful to divide the year into 90-day increments. Provide training to leaders each quarter, and include a "state of the union" address about the status of the organization's progress toward key goals, an update on relevant issues in the operating environment that impact the organization, and skill-building sessions that directly relate back to closing those gaps.

How does all this relate to engagement? For one thing, this training should directly build the skill set of leaders to engage their direct reports, employees, and patients. Gallup has found that managers account for at least 70 percent of the variance in employee engagement. Skilled managers are the key to a culture of high performance.[10]

For another, leadership development itself is an important part of an engagement strategy for leaders. To be fully engaged, a leader needs to feel he is being developed...that the organization is giving something back that enriches him professionally. After all, engagement requires a feeling of competence.

In addition to feeling competent, for employees to fully engage, they need to experience a sense of meaningfulness and a sense of progress.[11] They also want a sense of choice (i.e., a clear purpose, trust, access to accurate facts and information) as we have discussed above.

The "Must Haves" are designed for engagement. Over the years, Studer Group has identified specific evidence-based practices that we find to be essential for sustained high performance. These are also highly effective for increasing engagement. We believe so deeply in the power of these practices that we refer to them as Must Haves®.

In fact, we intentionally developed practices to improve the healthcare experience for each of the three stakeholders in our mission: employees, physicians, and patients. To engage employees, the key must-have behaviors that facilitate engagement are part of a comprehensive and systematic approach to selecting and retaining talent.

When it comes to employee engagement, those practices have to start before that employee even joins the organization. In fact, one of the things that we've advised organizations to do is right out of our own playbook for hiring practices at Studer Group.

If you want to work at our organization, before you even get a job application, we send you a set of our standards of behavior. These are very specific guidelines—deeper than our values even—that explain the expectations we have about how you'll conduct yourself as an employee.

And you'll read in those standards things like not gossiping about coworkers. We ask you to sign and return those before you can proceed in the interview process. What's truly wonderful about this practice is that perhaps 10 percent of individuals who receive these standards of behaviors elect to not return a signed copy to us. Therefore, they do not proceed through the hiring process. They self-select out, helping us to avoid low performers on the job later.

Others of us read those standards and feel validated in our choice of employer. So standards of behavior are a great way to selectively identify good matches for our culture and values…the people who are more likely to engage in the kind of team we want to create.

The act of asking everyone to physically sign the standards and commit to upholding them is intended to reflect a commitment to the organization's values, mission, and vision. It's not about hiring a homogeneous group of people who act and think alike. We seek to create safe places to work where people feel valued, ideas are welcomed, and employees trust what their leaders are communicating.

(To learn more about standards of behavior and how to implement them in your organization, visit https://www.studergroup.com/e-factor/standards-of-behavior.)

Behavioral-based interviews also facilitate engagement in a powerful way because when you base a hiring decision on questions that address job and skill sets—like analysis, initiative, and communication, for example—the likelihood of hiring someone who is a great fit improves dramatically.

We also find that peer interviewing by a potential employee's new teammates facilitates the integration and acceptance of the new person by his or her team. Once the hiring manager has pre-screened acceptable candidates, he forwards them to three to six high-performing peers who are trained on how to use behavioral-based questions.

The goal of those interviews is for them to only assess the fit of those individuals with values and standards of the organization. It's the final hurdle to join the team. (To learn more about behavioral-based questions and peer interviewing, visit https://www.studergroup.com/e-factor/peer-interviewing.)

This accomplishes several things. There's an old phrase that nurses eat their young in healthcare. And it's not just on the nursing side of things! Frequently, when a new person joins a team, they talk about how they used to do things at the last place they worked, which can cause resentment by new coworkers.

There's a natural competition to look better than the new guy. But when you as a coworker help make the decision to bring that new person on, you have a vested interest in their success. It's also the first opportunity we have as an organization to show that we value the new employee's input...that we really do encourage that innovation we talked about during the hiring process and *want* their input and experience. It all goes back to banking the trust that builds engagement.

As a result, those first 90 days become a more positive experience, which facilitates the engagement of the new employee right away. She has the sense that "Not only is my boss looking out for me, but my peers are too." This helps her feel centered, focused, and ready to give discretionary effort immediately. This practice is so powerful that one of our partners, Hugh Brown, CEO of HCA St. David's Georgetown, refers to peer interviewers as "the guardians of our culture."

Re-recruitment Starts on Day One

Remember how we talked about the high costs of retention? Well, Studer Group teaches that re-recruitment begins as soon as someone is hired. Don't wait months down the road to think about developing talent. That's got to start on day one.

I remember when I first joined Studer Group. My wife and I had just made this big decision to take this job. We were excited, but also a little anxious since she'd have to leave her job so we could relocate from Texas to Florida. We'd have to sell our house, buy a new house, and start fresh in a whole new community. We hoped we were making the right decision.

That night when Julie and I went out for a celebratory dinner, we returned home to find a giant plant on our front porch and a note from Quint Studer and BG Porter welcoming me to the company and telling me how excited they were to have me.

That gesture may have cost the firm $100, but boy did it pay dividends in terms of my engagement. It validated that we'd made a good decision, joining a group of people who really cared about us. Between the time that plant arrived and I showed up at work, I was all in.

That's why we very intentionally teach this practice to organizations we coach. Recognition increases engagement. It's important to understand, however, that people prefer to be celebrated and rewarded in different ways. While the best forms of recognition are those that are very personal to their needs and interests, there are still some forms of recognition that everyone agrees have a huge impact.

At the top of that list? Handwritten thank-you notes mailed to an individual's home. The very best of these is when they come from a senior leader who thanks you on behalf of a manager who has shared your contribution with them. Think about the power of this approach in terms of engagement.

Imagine that Helen, a CNA, does a great job with discharge instructions for a patient and his family. Helen's supervisor notices and shares this with the CEO, asking him to send a thank-you to Helen. First of all, the CEO is happy to learn Helen's supervisor has trained her well on discharge education. Helen herself is thrilled to be recognized by the CEO, but even more importantly, she's been "re-recruited" by her direct supervisor. She feels valued, and their bond is strengthened.

And finally, Helen may even share her note with family members. She becomes a role model for others to emulate service to patients. I can tell you from my own experience that this is powerful indeed. If you want to connect me to the organization, I'm even more engaged when my family learns about my contribution.

I'm fortunate to receive these notes from time to time myself. Sometimes when I'm on the road, my wife, Julie, opens these thank-yous in the mail. When I'm gone for three or four nights, she has to do more than her share around the house and take on all of the responsibilities for our kids. It can be exhausting.

But when I arrive home at 10 p.m. with everyone asleep and see a thank-you note that she's read on the counter from a hospital CEO that thanks me for a talk that's re-engaged their leadership team, we are both reminded that what I do every day when I'm gone is sacred work that's worth the investment of our time and energy.

What's even more incredible is when she reads these notes to my kids. In fact, in my son's kindergarten class a few years ago, they asked the kids what their mom and dad do while they're at school. My son answered, "When I'm at school, my dad helps doctors and hospitals give better care to patients."

Do you know how great that makes me feel? I even shared what he wrote with my mom: "You've always wondered what I do. Sam nailed it!" Then I came home and said to my wife, "Julie, that was so nice that you told Sam to write that."

And she said, "I didn't tell him to write it. I didn't even know they were doing this at school." So I asked her how he knew to use those words. She told me that she thought it was because it was the language he heard again and again in all those thank-you notes. Since he was born, that's what he's heard about my job.

Talk about engagement. That's a lot of mileage from a short note that took someone a minute or two to write and the cost of a postage stamp. Please don't miss this opportunity to re-engage people in your own organization. (To learn more about thank-you notes, visit https://www.studergroup.com/e-factor/thank-you-notes.)

The #1 Most Powerful Thing You Can Do

If you can do only one thing to improve engagement, make it rounding for outcomes.

It's an action-packed, evidence-based list of communication practices bundled together in a single 10-minute conversation once a month between a supervisor and direct report. And more than any other tool or practice that we prescribe, rounding for outcomes will profoundly move the metric of employee engagement and reduce turnover.

Why? Because it directly responds to the number one reason employees say they leave: a poor relationship with their supervisor.[12] What an employee wants most in a leader is approachability, to work "shoulder to shoulder," tools and equipment to do their jobs well, appreciation, efficient systems, and opportunity for professional development. These desires are highly correlated to the 12 questions that Gallup asked 80,000 managers in their 1998 landmark study to determine drivers for productivity, profitability, employee retention, and customer satisfaction.[13]

In fact, rounding for outcomes is an excellent way to engage millennials in particular. On the one hand, some say that millennials are narcissistic, self-centered, and only interested in a job as a stepping stone to the next job. (This is the first generation that was getting trophies no matter how many games their soccer team won at the end of the season.)

On the other hand, we know that millennials have a greater need for a sense of meaning in the work that they do when compared to other generations, and that they've been shaped by shared experiences like 9/11 during their formative years. They prefer to work as part of teams and like lots of feedback for development.

Personally, I'd take a team of millennials any day...and rounding for outcomes is a great way to engage them because it directly meets their needs for a personal connection, understanding the importance of what drives their work, and consistent, specific feedback. (Mostly, I like rounding for outcomes because it's about finding out what matters to John, the 25-year-old, rather than other tactics that assume the same things matter to all people who are the same age as John.)

How does rounding for outcomes work? First, a quick word about what it is *not*. It's not a quick "how's it going?" type of chat or "drive-by." Rounding is an intentional, scheduled activity designed to elicit specific actionable input.

There are just a few questions to ask when you round: (1) An opening question to build the relationship (e.g., "How is your family?" "Did your daughter's recital go well?") (2) "What's working well?" (3) "Is there anyone who has been helpful to you that I can recognize on your behalf?" (4) "Do you have the tools and equipment to do your job?" (5) "What systems or processes could be working better?" and (6) a question to ensure that key behavior standards in the organization are hardwired (e.g., "Tell me how you're explaining the role of the residents to our patients.").

In fact, if you were so keen to develop a revolutionary employee engagement tool that you commissioned a research study to do a meta-analysis of all the data that's published in management and psychology literature—the very best ways to engage employees—and then you distilled it down to a powerful set of practices that could be manageably added to a busy leader's plate, you would likely come up with rounding for outcomes.

That's just what we've done. For example, why do we start with a personal connection before we jump into the other questions? Because part of being an engaged employee is having a direct connection with your supervisor. It's all about that relationship. People join organizations; they quit bosses. If you want to get that Healthcare Flywheel spinning, it starts with having a stronger bond between supervisors and direct reports.

Often we're asked, "What if I don't know enough about them outside of work to establish that personal connection?" Well then, the first step is to learn something. This is not a fluffy strategy. If you want to engage people to do the things they're supposed to be doing, the biggest lever you can pull is the one that establishes a personal connection...that makes an important deposit in their emotional bank account.

If you're not sure what to talk about outside of work, or you feel the conversation getting stale, ask: "Where do you see yourself in three to five years?" This demonstrates to the employee that you're invested in them and their development.

The second question, "What's working well?" is next because it's important to acknowledge what's right before asking about what's wrong. If you've ever had the experience of walking around asking people about what could be better, you know that it encourages a negative response without many proposed solutions.

Frankly, that's just not a fun way to lead...Instead, identify ways to build gratitude and resiliency into your team. There's always something good you can focus on. Remember, it's hard to hold gratitude and bitterness in your heart at the same time.

The third question, "Is there anyone who has been helpful to you that I can recognize on your behalf?" is how you can harvest the opportunity for those thank-you notes that we discussed. Why? Because what gets rewarded gets repeated. As a supervisor, this helps you build bridges…not just between you and your direct report, but also between them and their peers. Strong, collegial relationships improve engagement.

The reason we ask, "Do you have the tools and equipment to do your job?" is because having what you need to do your job is a prerequisite to engagement. Earlier, I shared that engagement requires satisfaction, competence, and willingness. You certainly won't feel competent if you lack the basic tools, systems, or processes to support the outcomes you're being asked to produce.

In my job, I need a laptop, phone, and the assistance of my colleagues to feel competent. Those are the tools I need. Otherwise, it's hard for me to feel engaged. You want to be proactive in removing any barriers, whether they are small irritants or big issues. And this rounding question accomplishes that.

And finally, close by verifying that whichever behavior standards your organization is focused on improving are hardwired in that department. Why? This protects the culture of engagement you're building. It's not enough for new employees to commit to following standards of behavior. They must continue to be role modeled by everyone else consistently. (To learn more about rounding for outcomes, visit https://www.studergroup.com/e-factor/rounding-for-outcomes.)

And finally, follow up, follow up, follow up! If you're going to ask employees for input but not close the loop on what they tell you, you shouldn't be rounding at all. In fact, the best way to damage a relationship is probably to ask somebody for feedback, hear it, and do nothing with it.

> **The best way to damage a relationship is probably to ask somebody for feedback, hear it, and do nothing with it.**

That destroys a relationship. The key to the round is the quality of the follow-up, so make it a priority. One of the best ways to hardwire follow-up from rounding is through the use of Studer Group's stoplight report.

The report tracks all the requests and barriers individuals shared and assigns them a status of green (complete), yellow (under review), or red (can't complete at this time and here's why). Collecting the wins for removing barriers and having an adult conversation about those you can't change are critical to building the trust that underlies engagement in the workplace. (To see a sample stoplight report, visit https://studergroup.com/e-factor/stoplight-report.)

Re-recruit Your High Performers

Re-recruit your high performers, develop your middle performers, and take an "up or out" approach with your low performers. (In fact, if you are experiencing areas of non-performance or poor outcomes with an employee, ask yourself if it's a "will" or a "skill" issue. The answer leads you down different paths for solutions.)

Earlier, we talked about the importance of objective measurable goals that define the results of leaders. One of the questions we often hear at Studer Group is: "If goals are objective and measurable, can't someone get a great evaluation who is still rude to colleagues or otherwise hard to work with? Is that fair?"

Here's how that's addressed: While year-end evaluations focus 100 percent on measurable results, mid-year reviews focus 100 percent on adherence to organizational values and standards of behavior. We call these individual reviews highmiddlelow® performer conversations.

Our goal with these conversations is to retain high performers, improve solid performers, and to set clear expectations for low performers about what they must do differently to remain on the team. Throughout the organization, we want to intentionally and systematically address each of these groups with these goals in mind.

How does this tie to engagement? It's obvious when it comes to high performers. Imagine that you hear your supervisor say, "Thank you for the excellent work you do. It's my goal to re-recruit you to the organization and develop an individualized action plan to make sure I understand what's important to you." Your level of engagement just went up.

Conversations with solid—or middle—performers provide you with one of the key elements of engagement: professional development. By sharing what's working well and demonstrating a vested interest in their success and development opportunities, solid performers are inspired to re-engage.

The goal of the low performer conversation is not to terminate them. Rather, the goal is to create an environment that encourages them to change. As we've discussed, you can't change anyone, but you can create an environment that encourages the person to change. And low performer conversations can facilitate that decision to change.

Sometimes, when a low performer hears objective facts about ways in which their performance and behaviors don't match the values, mission, or vision of the organization, they see the light. In fact, we've found that about one-third of people who receive this direct coaching do, in fact, improve.

The other way low performer conversations can help is to engage their co-workers. If that low performer chooses to exit, or their employment is terminated because they refuse to change, the rest of the team is appreciative that the organization refuses to tolerate individuals who don't live its values and standards, even if they get good results.

No one wants to work shoulder to shoulder with someone who consistently doesn't pull their weight. By addressing low performers, we are increasing the engagement of middle and high performers.

As you can see, engagement is not just a vague, aspirational concept. Rather, there are disciplined Evidence-Based Leadership behaviors you can apply systematically to ensure it flourishes in your workplace. While the communication tools included here represent those with the greatest impact on engagement, they are by no means an exhaustive list.

Frequency of communication, the use of multiple channels for communication, and the ways in which we communicate expectations all make an important difference. To truly engage employees, always err in favor of *more* rather than *less* communication.

Employee Engagement: What Wrong Looks Like

Rachael's first day on the job as a new registration clerk at Community Hospital was a little stressful. She'd left her old job (even though they'd offered her more money as their best clerk) because she was looking for a new challenge. But her new coworkers weren't exactly excited to be interrupted with all her newbie questions. In fact, one even rolled her eyes when Rachael had explained a quick registration process that had saved the team at her last hospital lots of extra time.

After a few weeks on the job, she wasn't sure she wanted to stay. One of the biggest problems was Bill, a clerk the patients really seemed to like, but Rachael found him lazy and late all the time. Not only that, but he had a habit of leaving his empty soda cans at the workstation she shared with him, which didn't seem very professional to her.

Her boss, Tina, seemed nice enough so Rachael tried to approach her about the problem with Bill. But in the end, Tina looked vaguely uncomfortable, smiled a lot, and talked about how great Bill was with patients. When Rachael got back to her desk and saw an empty soda can sitting there, she made a mental note to call her previous hospital and see if there was still time to get her old job back.

Employee Engagement: What Right Looks Like

Before Rachael was interviewed for a position as a registration clerk at Community Hospital, they asked her to read and sign a document to agree that she would comply with the hospital's standards of behavior. *Impressive!* she thought when she read about their no littering policy and how everyone was expected to make eye contact and greet coworkers in the hallways. *They seem really serious about making the hospital a great place to work.*

At the interview, her potential new boss, Tina, asked her to share some examples of how she handled difficult coworkers and patients in the past. She seemed pleased with Rachael's proactive approach to problem-solving and asked her to come back and meet with three people she'd be working with for a second interview.

During the peer interview, Liz, who was also a registration clerk, was particularly friendly and asked some insightful questions to see if she was a team player. Rachael liked Mario too. They established a nice rapport right away, and she was looking forward to working with him.

On her first day, she was surprised how relaxed she felt even though she had a million questions. Liz and Mario really went above and beyond to make sure she had a great day. So when Tina stopped by at the end of the week to round on her, she had lots of good things to say.

She asked Tina to send a thank-you note to Liz for spending part of her lunch hour training her on the registration system and one to Mario for coming to her rescue with a difficult patient when it was clear Rachael didn't have all the answers.

When Tina asked her if she had the tools and equipment to do her job, Rachael said yes, but she also shared a new approach for quick registration she'd used at her old hospital. Tina seemed really interested, which made Rachael feel like she'd made an important contribution in her very first week. When she saw it listed on the stoplight report as "implemented" a week later, she smiled to herself. *What a great boss!* she thought.

And she confirmed her initial impression shortly later when she learned Tina had just fired Bill, a coworker who was chronically messy and late. Apparently, he'd been reminded several times that he wasn't complying with the standards of behavior he'd signed, but he hadn't changed. Everyone else in the department was friendly, considerate, and efficient, and they were all ecstatic that they wouldn't have to put up with Bill anymore. Rachael congratulated herself on making a great decision when she chose Community Hospital.

Key Learning Points: Engaging Employees (A Requisite for Leaders)

1. Engaged employees avoid work arounds to deliver greater clinical quality and safety to patients.

2. High employee engagement reduces costly turnover.

3. Connecting to passion, purpose, and worthwhile work is at the very foundation of high employee engagement.

4. Studer Group's Evidence-Based Leadership framework—aligned goals, aligned behaviors, aligned processes—is designed to increase employee engagement.

5. Effective tools include objective leader evaluations, leadership training, and Must Haves such as behavioral-based interviews, peer interviewing, standards of behavior, thank-you notes, rounding for outcomes, and highmiddlelow performer conversations.

CHAPTER 5

Engaging Clinicians

If trust is at the heart of patient engagement, then the people who are on the front lines of delivering care have the biggest role to play. In healthcare, it's a team sport. From nurses and physical therapists to medical assistants and case managers, there are dozens of professionals who have an important impact on the engagement of patients and families.

For our purposes, though, I'd like to focus on the specific nuances of engaging physicians, given their unique relationship to the organization and the patient. While some physicians are employed, others are independent...and there are many unique arrangements along this continuum, each with their own benefits and challenges when it comes to engagement.

The important point is that while these strategies are geared to physicians, I urge readers to consider ways to apply and adapt them to the broader caregiving team. There are many!

Engagement Is an Antidote to Burnout

Physician burnout is expensive in many ways, but particularly with respect to financial costs. In 2013, average annual physician turnover was estimated at 6.8 percent.[1] Just think for a moment about the cost of this physician turnover to an organization. When you add in the costs of recruiting, start-up, and lost revenue generation, the cost to replace a single employed physician often exceeds $500,000.[2] And that's excluding fees for sourcing and advertising, interviewing, moving, and signing bonuses.

The good news: Engagement is a powerful antidote to burnout. To avoid these costs, work to build relationships and create an environment conducive to engagement. By creating a functional and positive workplace, we allow physicians to maximize their effectiveness, no matter how simple or complex the case.

An experienced physician can become bored by too many routine cases that can be managed by advance practice providers. And yet, it's also important to be mindful about the consequences of loading up a physician with too many of those complex cases.

I remember one particularly poignant example shared by the leader of a successful telemedicine program focused on connecting emergency medicine physicians with rural hospitals through audio and video technology. While there were many benefits of this arrangement—enabling better care in the most precarious situations—an unanticipated negative consequence came to light when one of these physicians experienced four pediatric deaths in a single day. That's a burden none of us are prepared to shoulder.

If a clinician sees only the sickest patients, a high failure rate can trigger burnout by leaving him feeling discouraged and lacking that sense of purpose that's so critical to engagement. Conversely, when you effectively engage physicians in a partnership that truly serves them, the organization, and the patient, you mitigate burnout and create loyalty your competitors just can't beat.

And that's an important competitive advantage at a time when demand for physicians is expected to outpace supply substantially over the next decade. Engagement drives a sense of ownership that yields dividends again and again.

The Top Four Barriers to Physician Engagement

What disengages physicians? One study of physician burnout by the Agency for Healthcare Research and Quality (AHRQ) identified four problem areas.[3] The first is time pressure, the stress that results when there isn't enough time to see patients.

The second is a lack of work control, when a physician doesn't feel he has enough influence on his workplace or schedule. The third is the workplace itself, where inefficiencies, process breakdowns, and lack of tools detract from an effective work setting. And the fourth is the degree to which a physician's values and purpose aligns to that of the organization and its leaders.[4]

As you can see, it's important to understand what drives or engages a particular physician. Everyone has a different experience with these four areas. What seems like too much chaos to one physician might be an environment where another one thrives. To some degree, it depends on the individual.

Another survey by QuantiaMD also describes "de-motivating behaviors" for physicians with respect to their leaders.[5] Number one on the list—cited by 75 percent of the respondents—was leaders who weren't honest about the reasons behind their decisions. That was followed by "making promises but not delivering," "platitudes and vague business concepts," "expecting compliance without questioning," and "talking *at* me, not *with* me."

So what's wrong with asking physicians to comply with something you've organized for the greater good of the organization? For one thing, physicians want to understand the evidence for the change. That's what they do all day in evidence-based medicine. They wouldn't be skilled physicians if they didn't scrutinize the evidence for best practices, right?

Physicians Are Keen Observers

Physicians are keen observers by nature. In their patients, they look for patterns of health and disease. In their leaders, they look for evidence that they can trust them to create and sustain a practice environment that supports efficient and quality care. In other words, they seek Evidence-Based Leadership[SM].

Earlier, in Chapter 2, I shared five drivers for physician engagement: quality, efficiency, input, appreciation, and responsive communication. If you read up on this topic, you'll find it's a common theme. The QuantiaMD survey I noted above also identified "motivating behaviors" that echo this list. The top findings are open, honest communication; opportunity to be involved in decisions that affect me; being trusted to make decisions; and supported with resources.[6]

Essentially, physicians want to know their patients and family members are receiving high-quality care, even when they aren't there. They want their time demands respected through efficient operations so that their relationship with the organization doesn't feel like an impediment to their work-life balance and efficiency.

They appreciate an opportunity to provide a little input on how key work processes that affect them and their patients are implemented and operated. And, while they never say it directly, we all appreciate recognition and appreciation. Even physicians.

In spite of their long hours, physicians just don't go home at night to a mailbox full of grateful letters from patients, teammates, and administrators. In fact, frequently, those in the greatest positions of authority receive the least recognition and thanks. That's just one reason why thank-you notes go so far with them.

If there's just one thing that you focus on to facilitate engagement with physicians, it ought to be responsive communication. The bedrock of effective relationships is always trust and communication. Knowing a physician as an individual and forging a personal connection fosters that. Surprising our physicians with changes that impact them never does.

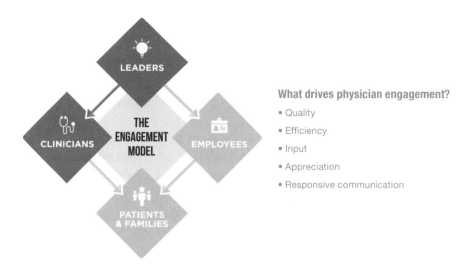

Figure 5.1 | Understand the keys to physician engagement.

You know who really gets this concept? Marriage counselors. A few years ago, I was facilitating a communication workshop and a chaplain in the audience who did some marriage counseling on the side explained how dismayed he was that it always came down to this same root issue with couples: communication.

So one day, when he was retiling the floor during his kitchen remodel at home, he got a bright idea. He brought a piece of the tile into his session the next day and said to the couple, "When I hand you the tile, you have the floor. As long as that's in your hand, you get to talk and the other person must listen."

About 90 seconds later, the wife began to cry. She looked up with tears still streaming down her face and said, "You know, that's the first time my spouse has listened to me for that long uninterrupted…for as long as I can remember." Active listening is just so powerful.

The Thing We *Always* Forget about Physicians

When you ask physicians to describe a great day at work, they will talk about days when they're not putting out fires or dealing with all the frictional costs of practicing medicine or administrative burdens. But even *more* notably, those best days occur when they make a powerful connection with a patient or a big impact on his health.

Never forget that physicians are driven by a sense of purpose. Maybe a challenging prognosis resolved well. Perhaps Mrs. Smith, who Dr. Fiorini has seen for the last 20 years, came in and said she's doing a little better managing her blood sugar lately. Those moments where a doctor is face-to-face with a patient making a difference is what got her into medicine in the first place.

And just like the Healthcare Flywheel® analogy demonstrates, connecting back to that sense of need for purposeful, worthwhile work that makes a difference in the lives of others creates more momentum for engagement. Be intentional in your organization in celebrating these moments both privately and publicly with your physicians. Don't let them filter out the positives of the sacred work they do every day. Help them stay connected to the difference they make in the lives of their patients.

Patients Are the Reason Doctors Went into Medicine

"The interactions I get with patients is the big part of my day. I get a charge out of having somebody sad who smiles; of having a kid who curls up on Mom's lap and refuses to have anybody look at them, but by the third visit is giving me high fives.

"It's good for my self-worth and my ego when I realize that I'm not the best surgeon in the medical group by far, but patients or parents will say, 'I want you to operate on my family. I want you to do this.' It's my interactions with them that make them want to do that."

—Otolaryngologist

Source: Janisse, Tom. "Relationship of a Physician's Well-Being to Interactions with Patients: Practices of the Highest Performing Physicians on the Art of Medicine Patient Survey," *The Permanente Journal*, Volume 12 no. 4 (2008): 70-76.

This holds true for most professionals actually. In fact, there was a *Harvard Business Review* study on engagement that asked software coders to track their level of engagement in their work daily, rating it from 1 (low) to 10 (high) each day and to write a few adjectives that described their day.[7]

They selected this group because they suspected they'd be hard to engage. Software coders operate on the fringe of our very virtual economy. They're frequently home-based, don't work in teams, and are very independent.

So what did they find? The days when these coders said they were most engaged weren't necessarily because anyone praised them. Rather, they felt an intrinsic sense of pride by advancing a task that they personally cared about on the job. Maybe they weren't sure how to write that tricky line of code at first...but hey, they did it!

High engagement also didn't happen on days when coding was easy. It could occur on a busy day...when the coders felt forward-focused, making progress on something they cared about. For our physician colleagues, nothing trumps time spent making an impact on the lives of patients and their families. Remember that. If your goal is to engage your physicians, create more opportunity here and remove the distractions to achieving this goal.

Myth-Busting about Physician Engagement

Here's the myth: "An employed physician is an engaged physician." It's just not true. There are many excellent reasons for health systems to employ physicians today, but assuming that employment will create engagement shouldn't be one of them. After all, you employ lots of other individuals. Are *they* all engaged?

There's an important difference, too, between physician alignment and physician engagement, two words that I find are often used interchangeably, which is a mistake. Just as I talked about how patient engagement is a higher order than patient satisfaction, so too is physician engagement a higher order than physician alignment.

Alignment is about matching organizational priorities, while engagement is about the discretionary efforts physicians give toward advancing the organization's mission. They're related, but not the same.

Think about it: It's really the difference between *compliance* and *commitment*. If a physician agrees to meet a quality goal set out by the organization, she's aligned. But will she give the discretionary effort to show she's committed to achieving it? Again, that's the definition of engagement.

In the same way, simply paying physicians for results is not an engagement strategy. While economic incentives can definitely be helpful in aligning a busy physician to the organization's quality agenda, it fosters alignment, but not necessarily engagement.

Physician Rounding 101

In the last chapter, I shared how powerful rounding with employees can be. (Note to our long-time readers: You may notice that as Studer Group® shifts to engagement, we are adapting language for rounding to replace "rounding on"—i.e., rounding *on* employees—to "rounding with"—i.e., rounding *with* employees—to better describe the partnership we hope to achieve.)

In fact, I said that if you could just do one thing to improve engagement, it should be rounding for outcomes. That holds true for building trust and a relationship as well. That's because it directly and positively influences all those key drivers of physician engagement we discussed a few pages back (e.g., quality, efficiency, input, appreciation, and responsive communication).

Your goal when you round with physicians is to demonstrate care and concern, harvest what's working well, give physician colleagues and direct reports an avenue to ensure their input is systematically heard and processed, ensure a mechanism to gain feedback about processes, and provide an opportunity to communicate with physicians about actions you are taking to make the organization a better place to practice medicine.

Here's how it works: Any leader—not just a senior leader, physician leader, or physician champion—can round with a physician…although these are the most common types of leaders we see round. Leaders who are responsible for the physician's work environment should be the primary rounders. That way, they can own the follow-up. It can also be helpful to assign executive team members to round with physicians. This helps everyone stay close to how his or her decisions are impacting physician engagement.

It also doesn't much matter whether the physician is employed, contracted, or independent (but some organizations do find it helpful for physician leaders to round with their employed physicians). The most important thing is to have a plan and to determine who would be most appropriate to round with whom based on the circumstances and organizational structure and then to cascade it down.

What about frequency of rounding? There's no single answer as every organization functions differently. It also depends on the role of physicians who are being rounded on as well as their impact (e.g., physicians responsible for high volumes).[8] In general, the more rounding the better.

If physicians are rounded on once monthly, physician engagement will be in the top 10 to 15 percent. If they're rounded on quarterly, engagement will be in the top 25 percent. If physicians are rounded on just once or twice annually, expect their engagement to be in the bottom 50 percent.[9]

When you round, you are going to use the very same questions used for employees, but adapt them slightly for physicians: (1) Focus on the positive ("What's going well today?"); (2) Harvest wins ("Are there any hospital staff or other physicians you feel deserve to be complimented or recognized?"); (3) Identify process improvement areas ("What systems can be working better?"); and (4) Repair and monitor systems ("Do you have the help and equipment that you need to care for your patients?")

It's useful to consider why the questions are ordered the way they are. It turns out there's quite a bit of science behind this approach. For example, by making a personal connection and starting with the positives, we've found it less likely that these sessions turn into complaint sessions with a long list of frustrations to be solved.

Here's the amazing thing about rounding with physicians: Even though you've been girding yourself for difficult conversations about things like requests for greater compensation and adding a new surgical wing to the hospital, you'll likely find that the typical concerns physicians express are far easier to fix.

When physician leaders at Ochsner Health System in New Orleans, Louisiana, began rounding, for example, the issues that came up were daily annoyances. One physician said the lock on the door didn't work and he'd been asking for it to be fixed for two months, but couldn't get approval to buy a new lock.

Another explained that she had to walk to the other side of the building every time she needed to print something out for a patient because she couldn't get a new printer. As a result, there were lots of early wins that leaders could communicate back quickly during their rounds. And that's what builds engagement.

But if you do hear things that can't be addressed, here are a few tips: First, if you know the answer is going to be "no," share that upfront and explain the reason why. The "slow no" undermines your informal authority, while a sincere and direct "no" with a solid rationale can earn respect.

Second, if something is asked for that can't be achieved without significant resources or time, learn to reframe the question. An example: "I understand that you're concerned about the current EHR and I'm glad you have some ideas that would help. I'd like to connect you with John, who is charged with identifying and remedying exactly these types of issues. I also understand that the fix may take some time. Given that, *what can I do for you this week* that would help you feel more engaged with the organization?"

Next, document the round so you can track follow-up and the physician knows you are committed to following up on issues he or she raised. Use Studer Group's stoplight report as explained in Chapter 4. If you end up with a long list of issues raised by physicians, ask the formal medical staff leadership to prioritize them. Then communicate this list to physicians and consistently re-communicate your progress on addressing the issues. Remember, communication drives physician engagement. (To learn about Huron's electronic MyRounding® tool, which also offers instant access to trends and issues that are identified, visit https://www.studergroup.com/e-factor/my-rounding.)

A tip to maximize the success of rounding with physicians: Build your own engagement in this process by always beginning with the physicians you perceive as most engaged and enthusiastic about change. This will build your confidence.

Then move through your list, saving the most challenging physicians for last. The reality is that your physicians will tend to fall into a few groups. The ones who are already loyal and the group who want to be engaged (but are held back due to a single issue) are going to be more rewarding to round with than those who are skeptical with lots of concerns and the group who will never get on board no matter what you do. Put your energy where it matters most—with the physicians you can influence and engage. (To download Studer Group's physician quadrant exercise, visit https://www.firestarter-publishing.com/e-factor.)

Other Ways to Get Physician Input[10]

While rounding with physicians is highly effective, it's not the only way to find out what's on the minds of your physicians. For instance, focus groups have been used in healthcare for years. They add value as the group setting can trigger ideas that might otherwise get lost.

Physician engagement surveys can also be a great way to gain more insight into how physicians feel about specific services (e.g., emergency, pathology, surgery) in a health system. Think of the survey as a diagnostic tool for physician engagement—like an MRI or CT scan. The data pinpoints where to focus, where there are no issues, and which items to prioritize in addressing.

And finally, consider the "Day in the Life of a Physician" exercise. It's just what it sounds like: Each participating leader chooses a different physician to spend the day with on a normal workday. If a physician is going to the clinic, the leader meets with them there. As you might expect, many leaders return from their day saying, "I'm surprised they're not more frustrated than they are. I have some ideas on how to make things easier."

How to Identify Physician Leaders

Physician engagement doesn't happen on its own. Momentum really gets rolling when physicians lead physicians to create a critical mass of support for the organization's mission. These leaders drive engagement because they lead by example.[11]

Effective physician leaders are:
- respected clinically by their peers
- high performers who can influence others
- progressive students of change who understand differentiators in the marketplace
- collaborative by nature and consensus-builders
- excellent at communicating a vision and articulating a strategy to achieve results
- not slowed or distracted by individual protests that run counter to the group's mission
- individuals who depend on measurement—not opinion—to assess performance

Selection criteria also include:
- high peer respect
- positive patient feedback
- relentless commitment to be the best

Hiring (and Keeping) Great Physicians

In the past, organizations have traditionally concentrated on clinical competence when hiring physicians. But today, that's not enough to predict the success of a physician. In fact, when it comes to creating engaged patients, it's critical that physicians have strong interpersonal skills.

It's also important that you choose physicians whose conduct, behavior, and clinical performance is consistent with your organization's standards and aspirations. And some of the best judges of that are the prospective candidate's physician peers.

That's why peer interviewing is so valuable. Recently, at Studer Group's annual What's Right in Health Care® conference, I heard a speaker from HCA, Hugh Brown, CEO at St. David's Georgetown Hospital in Texas, talk about peer interviewers as the "gatekeepers to culture." It's just so true.

As peers, physician colleagues are uniquely qualified to assess a fit between the candidate and the organization. While employed physicians and community physicians may look through different lenses, including both in the interview process creates a shared investment in the success of the new hire and the organization.

Here's how peer interviewing works:[12]

Select the physician interview team. Team members should include the medical director, department chair, and another physician who will work in close proximity to the candidate. The interview team should also include the dyad operational leader and a staff member who will work closely with the new hire.

Also, be sure to choose only physician interviewers who are identified high performers in the medical group. They must meet the standards of the group in attitude and behavior as well as clinical competence. They should also be individuals who are recognized as engaged themselves, modeling the values and standards of the organization and promoting the practice's culture (versus merely "sharing the load").

Use both behavioral-based and skills-based interview questions. Ensure that the interviewers you select are willing and able to participate in a two-hour training course on how to use behavioral-based questions. These questions are divided into two categories. The first—behavioral-based questions—seek information about prior conduct in specific situations (e.g., "Describe a situation in which you and another physician with whom you worked did not get along. Tell me about that situation and how it worked out."). These questions focus on teamwork and collaboration, caring and compassion, communication, leadership, and judgment/problem-solving.

The second set of questions—which focus on a theoretical situation—are designed to give the applicant an opportunity to express knowledge and opinion about a presented scenario. They analyze competencies in six dimensions of physician performance, which range from professional competence to team relationships.

To learn more about Studer Group's recommended physician selection process or to review examples of effective behavioral-based questions that address core organizational values and the six dimensions of physician performance, see an excerpt from the Physician Selection Toolkit at www.firestarterpublishing.com/e-factor.)

Assessing Engagement in Prospective Physicians

Remember Dr. Judith Hibbard's research on using Patient Activation Measure—or PAM scores—that we discussed in Chapter 2? She has also published several papers that examine the role of physician beliefs about the self-management of patients and the effect those might have on their patients.[13, 14]

While Hibbard herself admits that she initially thought all physicians would likely be in favor of more activated patients, she was surprised to learn that just wasn't the case. In a 2009 study to assess clinician beliefs about patient self-management, she adapted questions from her Patient Activation Measure questionnaire to physicians and found that it reliably measures how the physician views their role in the care process.[15]

The findings: While clinicians who were surveyed strongly endorsed the practice of patients following medical advice, they were less likely to believe that patients should make independent judgments or take independent actions. They were even less enthusiastic endorsers of patients functioning as a member of the care team or seeking out information independently. This is a real problem in an era where we need to empower patients to do just that if our organizations are to be successful in the era of value-based care.

Fast-forward to another study by Dr. Hibbard and her team in 2016 where they examined the role of primary care providers (PCPs)—physicians on the front lines of care—in patient activation and engagement in self-management.[16] The results? PCPs who had patients with PAM scores that were going up were much more likely than those with PAM scores that were flat to engage in supportive self-management and patient behavior changes…things like agenda-setting, problem-solving, and working in partnership with doctors to set goals. In fact, there was a positive correlation between PCPs' beliefs about patients' ability to self-manage and the actual improvements in their patients' level of activation.

> **PCPs who had patients with PAM scores that were going up were much more likely than those with PAM scores that were flat to engage in supportive self-management and patient behavior changes.**

Clearly, this has important implications for physician selection. In fact, according to Dr. Hibbard, some organizations are using physician CS-PAM scores (clinician support for patient activation) as a hiring criterion to choose physicians who are more engaged and therefore better aligned with the industry's shift toward the self-management required of patients under population health.

How to Train Physician Leaders

Now that you've selected physician leaders, what's next? Effective physician leadership skills weren't taught in medical school, so you'll need to use books, case studies, retreats, and mentoring to help your physician leaders excel.

Or, if you want to access a ready-made blueprint for what works well, you can consider Studer Group's popular Physician Leader Development program. It's a 12-month program that drives the implementation of proven, evidence-based practices. (Learn more at: https://www.studergroup.com/e-factor/physician-leader-development-program.)

While there are more than 10 key competencies we teach, a few of the most important are to:[17]

- communicate your organization's vision of engaged physicians, employees, patients, and families
- employ specific clinician-patient skills to connect, demonstrate empathy, narrate, and coordinate care
- use the language of engagement to express the value of using tools like AIDET®, rounding for outcomes, individualized patient care, and teach-backs with patients
- role play using physician communication tactics to improve patient engagement
- link key physician behaviors and communication skills to the ACGME competencies of patient care, interpersonal skills, communication, and professionalism
- make the medical workplace a positive interpersonal culture and confront inappropriate behaviors

Physicians Need Systematic Performance Feedback

Once we've hired the best physicians, trained them, and developed them, we need to create a process of systematic feedback because it is also an important predictor of physician engagement, as we've discussed. What do I mean by systematic? Each person doesn't invent his or her own feedback process. Rather, it should be an objective process using the same framework that is hardwired into the organization's approach to measuring clinical quality for every physician.

Physician goals flow from organizational goals with individual goals and weighted metrics to clarify expected priorities. Then, progress is reviewed face-to-face with individual physicians at least semi-annually.

Be responsive. While physicians appreciate data, don't make the mistake of simply sending it over with a cover letter. If you're interested in physician engagement, be an engaged leader.

If you choose to share the data ahead of time, follow-up quickly thereafter with an in-person meeting where you can answer the inevitable questions that will arise on the spot and, most importantly, talk about what it means, why it matters, and collaborate to identify opportunities for improvement. Learn more about Studer Group's INVEST framework to connect and provide feedback at https://www.studergroup.com/e-factor/invest.

Don't let those questions and concerns fester. Remember, communication drives physician engagement, but only if there's ample opportunity for two-way communication.

Be relevant. Are you sharing patient data that's 18 months old? Or a sample size of four? That's not useful to a physician. Bring current data and, ideally, include performance measures endorsed by the physician's specialty. If you invent a terminally unique metric that's not recognized by the specialty, don't be surprised by a less than enthusiastic response.

Be balanced. When you think about how to weight various physician metrics, consider the scope and role of the physician. The goal is to give feedback that reflects the entirety of the role. Studer Group organizes these according to People, Service, Quality, Finance, and Growth. To learn more about Studer Group's Provider Feedback System℠, which is designed specifically to accomplish each of these objectives, visit https://www.studergroup.com/e-factor/provider-feedback-system.

Seven Tips for Getting Physician Buy-in on Patient Experience Results

Many clinicians have a difficult time understanding and analyzing patient experience reports. For clinicians, the reports are essentially "data rich, but information poor."

To provide this data to clinicians in a more meaningful way, consider these tips courtesy of my Studer Group colleague Dr. Jeff Morris:

1. Present a rolling 12 months of data. A trend is better than a snapshot of a negative or positive "blip."
2. Ensure an adequate sample size by excluding low "n" results that skew data, a common problem for data in surveys of short periods.
3. Present data by "service date" rather than "receipt date" to better identify trends and impact of interventions and/or changes.
4. Present limited data in a meaningful way. Focus on a specific element (especially in "high priority/high correlation" areas) that you are working to improve (e.g., "explained clearly" or "dignity and respect").
5. Offer resources and training that are proven to positively impact the specific element that you are working to improve.
6. Connect the dots. Link back to the *why* that is at the core of the patient experience, rather than focusing on the *score*. (Examples: enhanced reputation, greater market share, optimized reimbursement, less liability, improved clinical outcomes, and less professional burnout.)
7. Sometimes less is more. Consider giving each physician a simple three-page report that is easy to decipher and practical to respond to: (1) question analysis, (2) priority index report, and (3) solutions to address the identified priority indices.

Grow Physician Champions

Perhaps the greatest opportunity for improvement related to physician engagement is to develop physician leaders into champions within the organization. Physician champions are excellent advocates and natural leaders of key projects and initiatives. Through their development, they become experts in the focus area (e.g., patient experience, performance appraisals) so that they can train, mentor, and build the skill set of their colleagues.

While some physician champions will have formal titles, others will not. But in both cases, they are invaluable in building the breadth, depth, and physician alignment within the organizations they serve.

Remember, too, that development is a key driver for physician engagement. Physician champions are physicians who are widely respected by their peers and are intentionally developed through specific leadership training to build systems and processes that make it easy for physicians to do the right thing at the right time across the organization.

Each of the tools I've shared here are powerful evidence-based approaches to dramatically improve physician engagement that have been time-tested at hundreds of healthcare organizations nationwide. And when you combine them together and apply them consistently over time, you build—and sustain—a world-class organization.

Physician Engagement: What Wrong Looks Like

Dr. Robbins was frustrated and exhausted. His clinical days had increased by several hours since ABC Health System had mandated new electronic health records. Not just that, but all that typing during a patient visit made it so much harder to connect with patients, which used to be the best part of his day. He was beginning to wonder how much longer he could do this.

Plus, it seemed like every day there was a flood of new emails about the latest organizational initiative to shore up reimbursement thanks to a new government regulation…or meetings he was supposed to drive to clear across town for some task force or to hear about the latest thing Administration had dreamed up to "improve patient care." When would they like him to do those things exactly? After he finished his 12-hour day? This wasn't why he got into medicine.

He was also awash in reports about his latest patient satisfaction scores, but ignored them, because, frankly, they were old and he didn't believe the data was valid anyway. The worst thing, though, was the little things that drove him crazy every day. He felt embarrassed every single time he walked into a patient room and asked a patient to sit in that rickety chair. He'd asked some-one to replace it three times, but they'd forget or say it wasn't in the budget or tell him they were still waiting to hear back. Why was that *so* hard?

Retirement was looking better every day.

Physician Engagement: What Right Looks Like

It's no secret that frustration with electronic health records (EHRs) is at the top of many physicians' lists of frustrating administrative burdens. But one medical group, ProHealth Care Medical Group (PHMG) decided to tackle that barrier to engagement head-on when physicians said inefficiencies and extra work for the EHR were causing burnout.

"I feel that fixing physician burnout is at least 70 percent organizational re-sponsibility," explains PHMG Chief Physician Operations Officer Brian Lipman. "If some organizations can reduce physician days, shouldn't that be our goal too? Why should the clinical documentation in EHRs require an additional three hours of the physician's day?"

The solution: a fun and supportive training session designed to speed adop-tion by making changes to each physician's personal configuration of the EHR on the spot. Attendance was high because PHMG offered CMEs and multiple, convenient training times.

The result: Fully 83 percent of attendees said the program would improve their job satisfaction and 69 percent said it would reduce the time they were spending working on EHRs outside of normal clinic hours.

(At another Studer Group partner organization, members of the IT team shadowed physicians for a day to offer real-time suggestions on how to improve the efficiency of the EHR. They measure their success by the number of "clicks" they are able to reduce during each of a clinician's encounters with a patient.)

Key Learning Points: Engaging Clinicians

1. Engagement is an antidote to physician burnout.

2. Physicians want quality, efficiency, input, appreciation, and open, honest communication. They're driven by a sense of purpose and making a difference in the lives of their patients.

3. Physician rounding is a powerful way to build relationships with physicians. The goals are to demonstrate care and concern, harvest what's working well, ensure input is heard and acted upon, get feedback, and communicate actions you are taking to create a better practice environment.

4. Provide objective, systematic feedback to physicians on performance at least every six months.

5. Be intentional about growing physician champions in your organization to increase momentum for engagement organization-wide.

CHAPTER 6

Engaging Patients and Families

Now that you understand what engaged leaders and engaged physicians do, let's look more closely at how to engage patients and their families directly. So far, we've identified that engaged patients are "activated"; they accept responsibility and are accountable for their healthcare.

In Chapter 1, I also noted that engaged patients strive to be informed about their care, are involved in healthcare decisions, participate in self-care, self-monitor and provide information, provide feedback on their experience and outcomes, and commit to long-term lifestyle changes. These are our goals for engaged patients.

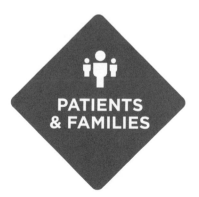

What drives patient engagement?

- Strive to be informed about health
- Are involved in healthcare decisions
- Participate in self-care
- Self-monitor and provide information
- Provide feedback on experience and outcomes
- Commit to long-term lifestyle changes

Figure 6.1 | Patient engagement is defined by six factors.

As we've discussed, physicians and other caregivers are the people who can best encourage patients to be accountable for their own healthcare. So let's consider next which tools and practices they can use to create an environment where these markers of engagement are likely.

While patient engagement is still a young science, particularly when we compare it to the decades of research we can access on employee and physician engagement, there are some emerging best practices we can rely on right now to better engage our patients.

Studer Group® recommends four main practices: (1) Build trust through expertise and empathy; (2) Individualize the care; (3) Empower and partner with patients; and (4) Celebrate progress together. Let's consider each of these next...

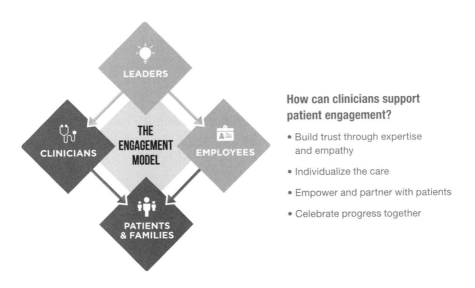

How can clinicians support patient engagement?

- Build trust through expertise and empathy

- Individualize the care

- Empower and partner with patients

- Celebrate progress together

Figure 6.2 | Use these four practices to support patient engagement.

Build Trust through Expertise and Empathy

Remember the old adage, "Nobody cares how much you know until they know how much you care"? It's true. Think back for a moment to the story I shared in the Introduction about my wife's experience at Highlands Rehabilitation Hospital during her dad's care there.

Remember how Victor sat down with Julie and her family and shared his own story of personal loss? He didn't view Julie's family as a patient ID number; rather, he took time to connect with her as a person. He embraced her as a fellow human being in the process of losing a father, just as he had recently. Nothing builds trust as powerfully as moments like these.

Who Are *Your* Patients' Heroes?

Remember how I explained in Chapter 5 that patient relationships are what drive physician engagement? Here's an example of how one executive at Mary Bridge Children's Hospital and Health Network in Tacoma, WA, used rounding to capture that win.

"When I asked a charge nurse where I should round, she directed me to oncology, where I found myself in a patient room with Jacob, a three-year-old little boy who was recently diagnosed with a rare pediatric cancer. His mom, grandparents, and an infant sibling were all present.

During the round, I asked if there was an individual team member deserving recognition for going above and beyond. Without pause, Jacob's mother said, "Dr. Reid. He's been so wonderful."

This surprised me because Dr. Reid wasn't part of the oncology team and hadn't played a role in either of Jacob's hospital stays. He is a primary care pediatrician who, coincidentally, reports to me. In fact, we were scheduled to meet for his performance appraisal the very next day.

Then she explained that while Jacob was in oncology, she herself had been admitted to the hospital a few days ago to give birth to his sibling. Dr. Reid knew that Jacob was hospitalized and his mom would be anxious to get discharged, so he expedited things. Then, when the baby wasn't gaining weight, the parents missed a follow-up appointment while caring for Jacob. So Dr. Reid stopped by to see them in the hospital to complete the office visit right there.

He assumed all of this would fly under the radar so he was shocked when I recounted the story to him the next day during his review. He was even more shocked when I handed him four VIP baseball tickets to express my gratitude for such an extraordinary commitment to compassionate care. Stories like these make patient rounding the highlight of my week.

—Stephen Reville, MD, MMM, Physician Executive for Network Development
Mary Bridge Children's Hospital and Health Network
Tacoma, WA

Patients and their families experience anxiety during healthcare visits for a number of reasons. Such visits are often unplanned and can be disruptive to their schedules. They sometimes involve pain and can have a serious financial impact. As a result, patient anxiety can result in poor listening, a failure to disclose important information, defensiveness, and a lack of follow-through on physician recommendations.

And yet, it's not enough for a patient to know his or her caregivers are caring. They also need to know they're in good hands. Empathy is wonderful, but competence is key. That's why AIDET® is so powerful. It's a structured communication process that addresses what patients say they most want from their caregivers: empathy *and* competence.

Fundamentals of AIDET Plus the Promise^{SM}

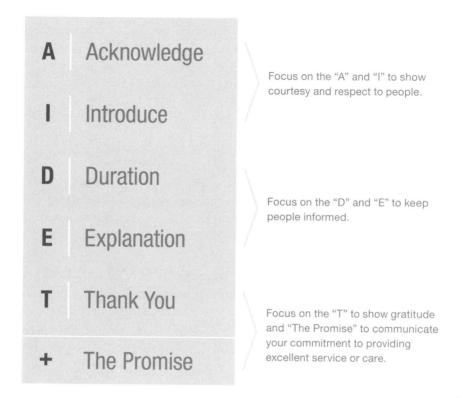

Figure 6.3 | AIDET Plus the Promise^{SM} is a powerful tool for patient engagement.

AIDET is not a script. Rather, it's a communication framework that builds patient engagement to improve clinical outcomes. If you're familiar with AIDET—Acknowledge-Introduce-Duration-Explanation-Thank You—you know it works in every department and discipline to reduce anxiety (for staff *and* patients). It ensures that caregivers consistently convey empathy, concern, and appreciation to patients *while managing up experience and expertise*. It's perhaps no surprise then that patients who experience AIDET are more likely to engage with their caregivers and follow medical advice.

The Promise recognizes that our patients are frequently frightened and worried when they seek our care and confirms their caregiver is committed to taking excellent care of them. From the family's perspective, they are comforted to know their loved one is in good hands. The Promise connects your heart to theirs.

Here's how AIDET Plus the Promise[SM] works:

A stands for Acknowledge. The key message here is: *You are important; I respect you.* Greet the patient by name, make eye contact, smile, and acknowledge everyone in the room with a smile, nod, or "hello." (There's even evidence for the importance of a sincere acknowledgment. In one study, 78.1 percent of patients wanted their physicians to shake hands while 91.3 percent wanted to be addressed by name.[1])

When it comes to increasing patient engagement, the "I" in AIDET is just so crucial. **I stands for Introduce,** as in, introduce yourself with your name, skill set, professional certification, and experience. Manage up yourself, co-workers, department, or organization in a positive way. (This helps "hand over" the trust that's earned with each interaction.)

Why is this kind of introduction so important? Because it responds directly to one of the most effective patient engagement practices that I mentioned above: It builds trust. The key message is: *You can count on me.*

Whenever I wonder about the power of the "I" in AIDET, I need only to think about my son Jack's experience when he had his first blood draw. He was five at the time. I don't know if you've ever taken a five-year-old to get his blood drawn, but I was a little anxious.

When I arrived, I chose a really wide chair so that he could sit next to me. In fact, I had my left hand around his chest, underneath his arms. My hand was right above his heart so I could feel it just pounding with apprehension. I was like his physiograph.

I know Jack pretty well, so when the phlebotomist laid out all the stuff she was going to use on him in line of his sight, I knew that was a big mistake. You want to hide that stuff!

So he's staring at this needle as the phlebotomist asks him the perfunctory safety questions: name and date of birth. She was nice enough. She told us her name was Ashley. But I knew it was time for some distraction.

So I said, "Hey, Ashley, just a question for you. How long have you been doing this job?" She said, "10 years." So I asked, "Do you work full-time doing this job?" And she nodded. "Like 50 weeks a year? Five days a week?" I prodded.

She said yes. So then I asked, "How many blood draws do you think you do in an average day?" She said, "20." So I did the math for Jack out loud: "Let's see…20 blood draws per day means you do 100 per week, which works out to 5,000 per year…or 50,000 blood draws over the past 10 years. Is that right?"

Ashley agreed she had probably done 50,000 blood draws. I could just feel Jack relax as his pulse slowed throughout our conversation. Jack knew he was in good hands. By introducing her experience, Ashley reduced Jack's anxiety and built his trust…the foundation for patient engagement.

Of course, Jack's blood draw went smoothly. Afterwards, I pulled Ashley aside to thank her and pointed out what a calming effect her words had on Jack. I suggested she share her expertise and experience with each of her patients before a blood draw to help reduce their anxiety and build trust.

Surgeons understand this. They're quick to tell you how many procedures they've done and what their complication and outcome rates are. They understand that patients face a very anxious moment when they have to make a decision to undergo a procedure…and that the credibility they bring will influence that decision.

But patients face lots of anxious moments when they interface with all kinds of caregivers, not just their surgeon. So why should only surgeons manage up their experience? Let's make sure that everyone does it. Be sure to hardwire AIDET in your organization with nurses, physicians, technicians, EVS, food service, administrators, and all staff involved in patient and family encounters at the bedside and across the continuum of care.

The D in AIDET stands for Duration. The key message is: *I respect your time.* Give the patient an accurate time expectation for tests, physician arrival, and identify next steps. When this is not possible, give a time in which you will update the patient on progress. Remember that "hope is not a strategy." Words like "hopefully," "as soon as possible," and "probably" undermine confidence and clarity.

The E stands for Explanation. The key message is: *I want you to understand so you feel safe and confident.* Explain step-by-step what to expect next, answer questions, and let the patient know how to contact you, such as using a nurse call button. Avoid jargon in favor of words the patient will understand and always offer an opportunity to ask questions after you explain something.

When I think about Explanation, I always remember my memorable experience at the eye doctor I saw when I was living in Dallas. I asked around and everyone recommended the same optometrist. What impressed me was that while she was examining my eyes and looking at them after they'd been dilated with bright light, she narrated her care. Instead of doing it silently, as is so often the case, she explained exactly what she was seeing. She'd say things like, "I'm now looking at the back of your eye and the vessels are opening up really well. It's very healthy. I love what I'm seeing here."

I learned about the anatomy of my own eyes that day. And I left thinking, *Wow! She's an incredible optometrist.* Was she incredible? I don't really know, but I do know she was a phenomenal communicator. And that ability to set someone at ease is part of being "clinically good."

This is called "competence by proxy." A patient can't actually assess the technical skill set of a surgeon, optometrist, or pediatrician. But he can *infer* it by rating the things that are visible or understandable. When a good communicator establishes trust and rapport, the patient assumes he or she is technically competent as well.

T is for Thank You. The key message is: *I want to provide very good service to you.* So a sincere thank-you shows appreciation and provides a positive close to the interaction. You could thank the patient for his courage or the family for their patience…or for being there to support the patient.

In fact, a statement of appreciation at any point in the interaction can serve to shift the dynamics of the discussion. When an ED physician says, "Thanks for being here to support your mom," during his first moments with a patient in the emergency department, anxious family members will feel reassured that their presence is valued. It builds that trust that is so crucial to engagement.

You might express gratitude to them for choosing your hospital or practice… or for their communication and cooperation. You could even ask: "What more can I do for you before you leave?" You get the idea. It's all about gratitude.

Add your Promise in the Introduction or Explanation part of AIDET. For example, say, "I promise to take excellent care of you today," or, "I promise to stay with you the entire time." When employees make that promise, their word becomes a bond they want to honor. Interested in learning more about how to hardwire AIDET? You can read more at https://www.studergroup. com/aidet.

Individualize the Care

As Dr. Hibbard, the patient activation researcher I mentioned earlier, emphasizes: The key to patient engagement is to *meet patients where they are.* That means that less engaged patients will need more help from their caregivers to become engaged while you can count on highly engaged patients to own the healthcare with less help from you.

In one study by Dr. Hibbard's research team, they identified five engagement strategies used by 10 clinicians whose patients had the highest PAM scores in that accountable care organization.[2] They learned that those whose patients had large increases in activation emphasized patient ownership, partnered with patients, identified small steps, scheduled frequent follow-up visits to cheer successes or problem-solve (or both), and showed care and concern for patients.

In short, they *individualized care to the needs of patients.* That's exactly what Studer Group's Individualized Patient Care is designed to do. It's worked effectively for more than a decade at hundreds of healthcare organizations to improve patient engagement.

Individualized Patient Care tracks organizational performance on what's most important to a particular patient—the *patient's* agenda—by asking, "What three things can we do to make sure your care is very good/excellent?" Those items should follow a patient—either through a piece of paper or in the electronic health record—through every encounter the patient has, from the check-in at the front desk to the medical assistant to the physician in a clinic setting.

In a hospital setting, the patient's responses are noted on a communication board in every patient's room. In fact, there's a special section on it that asks, "What's most important to you?" Then during daily patient rounds, the nurse manager checks in with the patient by asking, "How well are we doing with *(identified needs)*?" Individualized Patient Care is *not* what the plan for the day is!

Individualized Patient Care is also important in the outpatient arena. Imagine a parent who has been up all night with her child who has a fever. She brings the child in for care to the emergency department, but in the back of her mind what she's really hoping for is an antibiotic.

This may or may not be appropriate treatment, but if the clinician knows ahead of time what that parent really wants, he can reduce her anxiety so that she doesn't leave feeling her biggest concern wasn't addressed.

Ask: "What's most important to you during this ED visit?" It's a very important question and one that's quite different from: "What brings you to the ED?" While the fever brought the parent to the ED, her *expectation* is to get an antibiotic. This question works for the same reason in medical practice settings as well.

Keeping the communication board updated is critical. For Individualized Patient Care to impact patient engagement, there must be a communication board in every patient room *that is kept current.* Since the goal is to keep the patient informed, it should include the patient's goal, the next time medication is due, and anticipated discharge date and time among other things.

However, there is a caution to heed before you implement this practice: If you put up a communication board with lots of information and then you never update it, you will actively disengage your patients. Having a question on the board is like making a promise to meet their needs. If we fail to update it—or worse, update it once but never again—it is a promise broken.

Just imagine: You are lying there in the hospital bed and when the nurse leader rounded on you, you explained that you'd really like your sheets changed. You see that your next pain medication is due in two hours. But no one ever updates the white board so your request for clean sheets goes unanswered.

Family members become concerned when the nurse gives you your next dose of pain medication, but doesn't update the communication board. It starts to seem like a safety issue, so they begin updating it themselves. If you implement Individualized Patient Care, your staff needs to be all in. Keep the communication board current and accurate!

A quick side note: Studer Group finds that pre-shift huddles provide excellent opportunities to remind staff why it is so important to keep these boards current. Recognizing staff who consistently maintain up-to-date communication boards is vital. You can even encourage top performers to help their peers become consistent in this critical area of care delivery.

And remember, when nurse leaders round on patients (see "Verify with Nurse Leader Rounding" later in this chapter), they need to actively look for opportunities to observe staff doing a great job keeping communication boards current and be specific in their thanks. What gets rewarded gets repeated!

Little Things Mean a Lot to Patients

Still wondering about the power of Individualized Patient Care in engagement? Here's a story that long-time Studer Group partner and former coach Karen Fraser likes to share about it:

"While I was observing a nurse leader rounding with patients at one of our partner hospitals, I met a young female patient who was clearly very disengaged and unhappy. The nurse leader dutifully went through her list of specific rounding questions, and the patient provided her with one-word answers, never smiling or engaging in meaningful conversation.

"As the nurse leader was checking off her rounding log and ready to move to the next room, I decided to role model Individualized Patient Care with this young girl, in hopes that the nurse leader would learn, and, even more importantly, that this young patient's experience would improve.

"So I sat down next to her and gently explained how sorry I was she seemed to be so unhappy. I asked if there was anything we could do to better address her needs while she was here in the hospital. I explained that when people come into the hospital, it often feels as though they lose control of their daily lives. I let her know we were genuinely interested in knowing what things were most important to her while she was here.

"She looked up at me with distrusting eyes, but she took a chance and began to share her experience. She explained that at home, she liked to have fresh fruit with every meal. Eating a healthy diet was important to her. She said she had spoken with someone from dietary services about requesting fresh fruit with every tray, but several times she had to ask the patient care techs to call down for the fruit.

"Then she revealed something that made my heart sink. She said, 'I know they don't think I can hear them in the hallways, but I listen to every word they say. I'm so tired of hearing them make fun of my eating habits when it comes to fruit. I feel like my choices should be respected.'

"The nurse leader and I agreed wholeheartedly and we let her know how much we supported her choices and promised to do everything we could to make it right. I asked her what 'excellent care' meant to her.

"She said it would be wonderful to always have a set of fresh towels at her bedside so she could go take a shower whenever she chose to. She said it made her feel more independent and in charge of her own care.

"By now, I was standing up at the white board and capturing these simple, yet powerful requests. Lastly, she said, 'Would it be too much trouble to ask the staff to keep my door closed when they leave the room? This simple act makes me forget I'm in a hospital and makes me feel like it's really *my* room for as long as I have to be here.'

"Of course we agreed to everything and wrote the three things down on the care board in her room, which represented 'excellent care' to this young woman. By now, she was smiling, laughing, and fully engaged in the conversation. She hugged the nurse leader in thanks for listening to her desires."

This is the essence of what "engaging" our patients can look and feel like. Karen is such a passionate believer in Individualized Patient Care that she also likes to share her own story as a patient on the receiving end of such care. In November 2014, she developed a blood clot in her lower left leg that went undetected—because she was asymptomatic—until the following January, when the clot extended all the way up her thigh.

She was eventually referred to a vascular surgeon who offered her two options for her treatment plan: (A) do nothing through a conservative approach by continuing anticoagulant therapy for at least six months or (B) attempt thrombolysis of the blood clot via an inpatient procedure that would require two nights in the ICU, followed by option A.

But then, she said, her doctor did an amazing thing...something that she believes lies at the very heart of patient engagement. Her doctor asked what *her* long-term goals were in relation to healing from this blood clot. She explained that she very much wanted to return to normal activities as much as possible with minimum long-term side effects. She emphasized how important exercise was to her and that she hoped in time to get back to jogging a few times per week and lifting weights to keep her muscles toned.

Based on this feedback, her doctor explained why the procedure would be the best choice: The doctor would likely be able to dissolve most, if not all, of the blood clot, which would then make it possible to achieve Karen's goals. There were risks involved, which she explained in detail.

The doctor said she'd put Karen on the surgery schedule for Monday, simply to reserve a time slot in the OR. But she also asked Karen to go home and sleep on it and to call her over the weekend with any questions. She offered her cell phone number and said that "we"—the two of them—could decide before Monday morning.

Then she called to check on Karen Saturday and answered more questions. By Sunday, Karen was confident in the plan and called her doctor to let her know she was ready to move forward with the procedure on Monday.

Today, two years later, Karen has recovered extremely well. She wears a 30 mm compression stocking on her left leg whenever she's up and around because her doctor explained that the evidence shows this prevents long-term swelling in the leg that can be a typical side effect after a deep vein thrombosis.

At every follow-up appointment, Karen's doctor asks how she feels when she exercises or runs and wants to know if Karen feels she is achieving the goals she expressed early on. Karen gives her doctor bonus points for taking an extra moment to research the best brand of compression stockings to use for running through a quick online search during her actual office visit.

As you can no doubt tell, Karen is a loyal patient. Her doctor not only asked her what was most important to her, but she referred back to those things again and again in all of her follow-up care. She's got a patient for life. If you'd like to learn more about how to hardwire Individualized Patient Care in your organization, visit https://www.studergroup.com/e-factor/individualized-patient-care.

Hourly Rounding for Real-Time Engagement

The very best way to ensure that communication boards are being kept current with patient priorities, medication schedules, and discharge information is to update and verify it through Hourly Rounding® by nurses with patients. This every hour check-in with patients demonstrates our real-time commitment on an ongoing basis to delivering quality care to patients and engaging them directly in their own care for more ownership.

If you're not familiar with this valuable evidence-based practice, you can learn more at https://www.studergroup.com/e-factor/hourly-rounding. But here's a quick summary of the benefits: In 2006, Studer Group published a rigorous national study in the *American Journal of Nursing* that demonstrated Hourly Rounding reduces patient falls and pressure ulcers, improves patient satisfaction, and gives nurses back more time because patients use the call light far less frequently.[3]

One organization even credited Hourly Rounding with capturing $81,600 in annual lost charges.[4] They said the reduction in call lights was so dramatic that it created a calmer work environment for nurses. And as a result, nurses had more time to be proactive about documenting, educating patients, and attending to direct patient care needs.

While nurses who are unfamiliar with this practice may be skeptical about Hourly Rounding in the beginning, Studer Group's experience is that they quickly become believers. Again, if you do your job as an engaged leader when you roll out this tactic, connecting back to your organization's vision and mission and showing why it results in better outcomes, nurses will quickly engage.

As one CNO explained, "It creates an environment where our nurses have more time to do what they came here to do: provide the very best care to our patients."[5] Another tip for getting nurses on board is to document—and share with staff—the time savings that is actually resulting from fewer call light interruptions.

Verify with Nurse Leader Rounding

So let's say that you've implemented Individualized Patient Care and Hourly Rounding. How do you know that your nurses are actually using these tools with *every* patient *every* time? You'll use nurse leader rounding to verify that it is so.

Why wait on your HCAHPS survey results to find out that some patients didn't get rounded on or included in nurse shift changes? When nurse leader rounding is used consistently, leaders can manage the patient experience pro-actively, instead of learning later that a gap in care or expectations occurred through a complaint letter, poor outcome, or experience.

It's just what it sounds like: Nurse leaders round on patients to verify that appropriate care is being delivered by nurses. It's essentially a quality check. If there are gaps in care, the nurse leader then coaches the nurse in question rather than providing the care him- or herself.

Remember how we discussed the importance of empathy as a prerequisite for engagement? Nurse leader rounding communicates that "I am the leader and responsible for the quality of care delivered here. I care about you."

It also provides an opportunity for a patient to feel heard if service recovery is needed and to harvest reward and recognition of caregivers who went above and beyond. Remember, that's what fuels greater engagement for employees and physicians: recognition. To learn more about nurse leader rounding, visit https://www.studergroup.com/e-factor/nurse-leader-rounding.

The Power of Bedside Shift Report

One of the most effective ways of engaging inpatient or ED patients in their own care is through the use of the Bedside Shift Report. Even more potent is when Bedside Shift Report is used in conjunction with Individualized Patient Care during a hospital stay. Patients experience a strong sense that caregivers care about what's important to them and are invested in their speedy recovery.

Bedside Shift Report is effective because shift changes are a particularly vulnerable time for patients. We know it's a potential source of medical error. And it can be tough to say goodbye to a nurse a patient has bonded with. While he might feel anxious about that nurse's replacement, that's where Bedside Shift Report can help.

When it's done right, it's not about nurses talking together at the end of a patient's bed, in the hallway, or at the nurse's station. The shift handover includes the patient, manages expectations, provides training on medication or on a medical device, and validates the patient's understanding.[6]

Bedside Shift Report gives patients back a sense of control by bringing them into the care team. And, they frequently become more cooperative because they feel informed.

They feel they are partners in their care...that things are done *with* them instead of *to* them. Earlier, I explained that effective patient engagement strategies both empower patients and partner with them in their care. You can see how bedside shift report is a natural fit here.

At one of Studer Group's partners, Advocate Sherman Hospital in Elgin, IL, our coaching team recommended adding a custom question on the HCAHPS survey of patients to gauge the value of Bedside Shift Report: "At change of shift, did your nurses include you in the plan of care?" The results were astonishing.

The 600 patients who said they did ranked the hospital in the 85th percentile for HCAHPS overall rating of care, while the 76 patients who did not ranked them in the 1ˢᵗ percentile. The results here are clear: Patients who said they were included in the plan of care reported a better overall experience.

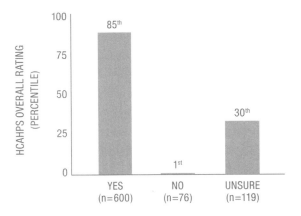

At change of shift, did your nurses include you in the plan of care?

Figure 6.4 | Bedside shift report makes a dramatic positive difference in HCAHPS overall ratings for patient care.

Source: Advocate Sherman Hospital, Jan to Mar 2016

Use the teach-back method during Bedside Shift Report to validate understanding. If you're not familiar with the teach-back method, it's essentially a strategy used by clinicians where they ask patients to explain back to them their understanding of what he or she is communicating, i.e., the diagnosis, the treatment options and recommendations, and how the patient intends to act on the information.[7]

It works in multiple care settings and is an excellent way for clinicians to assess what a patient has really heard and how "activated" he really is in terms of engagement. By assessing the information the patient shares during teach-back, a caregiver can then adjust his approach. If a patient didn't understand the diagnosis accurately or misunderstood the physician's instructions, information can be further explained.

For example, instead of asking the patient, "Do you know the side effects of this medication?" say: "I know we covered a lot of information. So that I can be sure I did a good job making this easy to remember, can you tell me some of the potential side effects of this medication that you will watch for and report?" This reinforces our expectation about what we expect a patient to do if a side effect occurs and allows us to further clarify if the patient isn't able to recall the side effects.

If the physician has some doubt about the patient's likelihood of following through with recommendations, she may choose to set a follow-up appointment sooner. Teach-back is such a valuable tool in allowing us to meet patients where they are on the engagement spectrum.

When clinicians and staff can see the evidence for themselves that a prescribed behavior makes an important difference in patient engagement and the overall patient experience, their values won't let them ignore it. Rather, they feel compelled to do it. Remember to always take time with your clinical care team to connect back to the evidence it works as you seek to achieve 100 percent consistency in implementing tools and tactics like these. To learn more about Bedside Shift Report, visit https://www.studergroup.com/e-factor/bedside-shift-report.

Engage Patients Before *and* After You See Them

When we consider ways to effectively engage patients, we need to think beyond the walls of our facility. Engagement isn't important just when they are with us in the clinic or hospital; it's also important both before and after the patient's appointments.

At Studer Group's 2016 What's Right in Health Care® conference, Warner Thomas, the president and CEO of Ochsner Health System in New Orleans, LA, shared his perspective on the value of pre-calls in his keynote address. He marveled at the fact that we already know which patients are most likely to miss or be late for an appointment.

In fact, one study conducted at Robert Wood Johnson University Medical Group, an outpatient medical specialty group, noted that more than 23 percent of patients who received no reminder call missed their appointments. That's expensive, both in terms of lost opportunity for improved health in the community and revenue to the organization. But they reduced the number of no-shows to 17.3 percent with an automated reminder and to 13.6 percent if an actual person called.[8]

JPS Health Network in Fort Worth, Texas, had a similar experience. On the one hand, they were averaging 100 days for next available appointments across some of their clinics. One culprit? A no-show rate that averaged 28 percent across clinics, leaving appointment slots unused but also unavailable. By adopting a multi-faceted approach that included pre-calling patients, it halved the no-show rate for a $1.3 million return on investment.[9]

But despite the fact that we have this data and know the appointment-missing history of such patients, we often fail to do anything differently to ensure they show up. These patients are likely less activated and deserve a differentiated approach to "meet them where they are."

That's where pre-visit phone calls to patients can be so valuable. When a patient misses an outpatient test or procedure, it puts their health at risk and also reduces access for another patient we could've seen. Don't let this happen in your organization. Pre-call patients at risk for missing an appointment.

Here's how they work: A basic pre-visit phone call confirms the appointment, explains the procedure, reviews instructions, provides directions to the facility, asks the patient to arrive early, and reaffirms the necessity of the visit.

Sample Key Words for a Basic Pre-Visit Phone Call

"Hello, Mrs. Smith, this is Sally from St. Vincent Mercy Medical Center. I am calling to remind you of your MRI appointment on Wednesday, July 6th. I see Dr. Smith ordered the MRI. He will be waiting for the results so he can update plans for your care. *(Many patients don't want to let their physicians down and will overcome their own resistance to the appointment when we frame the physician's expectation like this.)*

"Have you been to St. Vincent in the past? Do you need directions? Do you know where our MRI department is located? *(If not, give directions.)* If you can arrive 10 minutes early that will help us make sure the hospital runs on time for other patients. Is there anything else I can do for you today, Mrs. Smith? Thank you for choosing St. Vincent for your healthcare needs.[10]

"If for any reason you are unable to keep this appointment, please call us so we can serve other patients in the time we have specially reserved for you."

A "next level" pre-call also explains the patient's financial obligation, asks the patient to arrive prepared to pay their co-pay, and asks the patient to write down any questions for the doctor and bring them to the appointment. This type of pre-call will bring you a more engaged patient.

A Sample Advanced Pre-Call Also Includes:

"I see you are covered by Blue Cross-Blue Shield. Under the provisions of your 80-20 policy, there will be a co-pay on this particular procedure of 20 percent. The total cost is $1,000, so please come prepared to pay $200 when you arrive. That will take care of it so we won't need to bill you later. It will make things more convenient for you."[11]

One of the reasons post-visit calls have become even *more* valuable is that hospitals now face greater opportunity for both higher financial rewards and penalties under CMS's bundled payments rule, through which hospitals receive one payment for clinically defined episodes of care up to 90 days post-discharge.

By 2018, it's anticipated that 50 percent of contracts will be tied to alternative payment models like these...and 90 percent of contracts will be tied to quality or value overall.[12] You need to avoid readmissions if you want to avoid financial penalties under bundled payments, and that's where post-visit calls are useful. They keep you connected with patients after discharge. It's a safe bet that patient engagement will be the new core competency that is required for success under risk-based structures like bundled payments.

> **Patient engagement will be the new core competency that is required for success under risk-based structures like bundled payments.**

And really, is it too much for our patients to ask of us to check on them after they leave our clinic or facility? Perhaps you've seen the popular customer service training video *It's a Dog's World* by CRM Learning that contrasts the care that Bob the patient receives to that of his dog at the vet. While Bob gets treated like a dog during his doctor's visit—with long wait times and busy healthcare professionals—Bob's dog gets the royal treatment at the vet.

In fact, after Bob's visit, he hears his wife answer the phone… She says, "Oh hi, doctor. Thanks for calling. Yes, we filled his medications and he's resting fine. I'll let him know you called." But guess what? It's not Bob's doctor. It's the vet![13]

There's just no substitute for a post-visit phone call. The reality is that 19 percent of patients have an adverse drug event after discharge.[14] These calls allow you to prevent readmissions to the hospital by proactively addressing any potential clinical issues before they occur.

They extend care beyond the four walls of the facility. It's a powerful and effective approach to engage and activate patients between visits. You can use them to connect patients to care navigators, social workers, health coaches, nurses, and more.

Post-visit phone calls will always have a special place in my heart personally because I understand their value first-hand. My youngest son, Jack, was born a few weeks early. It was a scary moment, with the NICU team on stand-by since Julie had been induced so early. While Jack received top APGAR scores, his doctor was concerned that his breathing hadn't regulated—they were seeing some respiratory distress.

I watched Jack nearly constantly in the well-baby nursery from when they brought him in around 11:00 at night until probably 4:00 in the morning when I finally fell asleep. But then, two hours later, I learned he'd been transferred to the NICU, which was terrifying to hear.

Fortunately, the NICU was just 30 feet away from our room in the hospital that night. So I went over, scrubbed up, and went to Jack's bedside. There he was...hooked up to a lot of equipment. We were worried. (Although we really shouldn't have been. He was over five pounds...which makes him a sumo wrestler by NICU standards. In any case, he just needed to feed and grow.)

But just as terrifying as finding out Jack had to be moved from the well-baby nursery to the NICU was the moment when the team of neonatologists handed him to us to take home. I mean, one minute Jack required a whole team of specialists at a cost of thousands of dollars per day to keep him alive, and the next he's in our arms and they're giving us a folder of discharge instructions.

But then the physician said to me, "I know this is a lot to remember, Dad. So I want you to know we are going to give you a call tomorrow afternoon to check on Jack and answer any questions. Is 2:00 good for you?" I was so grateful that I literally teared up. What a relief...I truly felt I had a whole team supporting me that was invested in Jack's continued good health. Every patient feels this way after they get one of these check-ins.

A post-visit phone call is also a natural extension of the Individualized Patient Care you provided on-site to the patient at your facility or clinic. If you're tracking those top three patient priorities in the electronic health record, it will be easy to ask about them when you call the patient.

Checking in on what's most important to an individual patient after his visit is also an excellent opportunity to address and resolve any barriers to a quick recovery. So request that nursing staff and case managers ask, "How well have we done with *(identified needs)*?"

These calls also provide an important bonus: You can specifically ask if there's anyone who was especially helpful to the patient whom you can reward and recognize. It's another great way to drive employee and physician engagement. To learn more about post-visit phone calls or see a sample set of questions, visit https://www.studergroup.com/e-factor/post-visit-phone-calls.

A final note here: There's a number of ways to segment post-visit calls to improve patient engagement. And I predict that in no time, creative leaders will be using them to reach out to patients with low PAM scores, just as we have seen them reach out with a series of calls for more complex and readmission-prone patients.

In fact, Studer Group's Patient Call Manager™ solution makes it easy with features like serial calls for high-risk groups, color borders that flag patients who have been in your organization within the past 30 days, and other types of electronic triggers that allow you to maximize efficiency for a high-touch approach through personal phone calls to patients who need it most. To learn more about Patient Call Manager, visit https://www.studergroup.com/e-factor/patient-call-manager.

Empower and Partner with Patients

Engagement is all about empowering patients and partnering with them. It's no longer about what we do *for* patients; rather, it's what we do *with* patients. That's why information like Dr. Hibbard's research on the role of physician beliefs in the self-management of patients is so important, as we discussed in Chapter 5.[15]

To succeed at engaging patients, we *must* ensure that our caregivers and employees understand and share our belief that the role of the patient is important...we need them to understand that patients are our valued partners in making an accurate diagnosis, assessing a viable treatment plan, and ensuring a speedy recovery.

While you might think this is obvious, you need only to read the study about attitudes of primary care physicians that I just mentioned to understand the scope of the challenge. A surprising number of physicians today are out of step with the current direction of health policy, which urges patients to become independent actors with *support* by their physicians.

Such physicians frequently point to "time" as the main barrier to more shared decision-making. But in one review of 38 studies, there was actually no robust evidence to support this view.[16] Patient engagement cannot be optional in healthcare today...for anyone.

So what does patient empowerment and partnership look like on a practical level? It's all about communication. We've talked about how tools like Individualized Patient Care, Bedside Shift Report, nurse leader rounding, and pre- and post-phone calls address this. But perhaps the most powerful approach is the one used by an individual clinician with his or her patient during an office visit.

Teach-backs are excellent in this context. But I'd also like to share some specific strategies recommended by my Studer Group colleague Dr. Joshua Kosowsky, who literally wrote the book on this. Dr. Kosowsky organizes his recommendations into four areas: (1) Establish an active partnership, (2) Focus on the diagnosis, (3) Listen, and (4) Understand every test ordered. Please see the following chart for complete details.

Use These Four Strategies to Improve Communication with Patients

PATIENTS	PROVIDERS
#1. Establish an active partnership	
Set expectations	Set expectations:
Partner in your decision-making	• Be transparent
Ask to share in the thought process	Involve patients in the decision-making
	Explain your thought process
#2. Focus on the diagnosis	
Know why it is important	Explain why it is important
Ask for:	Provide every patient with:
• Most likely diagnosis	• Working diagnosis
• Other possibilities	• Differential diagnosis
Assure your doctor it's OK not to be 100% sure	
#3. Listen	
Tell a good story:	Really listen:
• Story, not symptoms	• "No questions asked"
• Begin at the beginning	• "With our whole being"
• Use your own voice	• Beyond the chief complaint
Come prepared:	• Will save time
• Write it down	Encourage preparation
• Practice	
• Bring an advocate	
#4. Understand every test ordered	
Ask about diagnosis before tests are done	Explain diagnosis
Understand why a test is being ordered:	Ask yourself, for every test:
• What is it looking for?	• How will it change management?
• What are the risks?	• Do I need it?
• What are the alternatives?	• How do I explain risks/benefits?
• What happens if negative?	

Figure 6.5 | Suggested Strategies to Improve Communication Between Providers and Patients During the Office Visit

Source: Reprinted with permission from *When Doctors Don't Listen: How to Avoid Misdiagnoses and Unnecessary Tests* by Leana Wen, MD, and Joshua Kosowsky, MD

Also, sit with patients whenever possible. Don't stand. When clinicians stand with patients, instead of sitting, they unwittingly send the message: "I'm busy." It takes only a few seconds to position ourselves in the proximity of the patient, but it makes a world of difference to a patient.

Here's why: It flattens the authority gradient between those who give care and those who receive it. And, while it takes no more time than standing, the literature shows that it also increases the perception of time spent by about 50 percent.[17]

In other words, when you sit, patients relax because you signal that you have time for what they might tell you. Therefore, they are more likely to speak up and provide feedback.

For years, much of the work on engaging patients in safety has been to ask them to speak up if something doesn't seem right. But in one study aimed at improving patient safety and reducing medical errors, where patients were asked about their level to ask certain kinds of basic questions, many patients were uncomfortable asking their clinician even basic questions like "How long will I be in the hospital?"[18]

So when it came to more challenging questions like "I don't think that is the medication I am on. Can you check please?" or "Have you washed your hands?" patients were very unlikely to speak up. But if patient safety is important, our patients must feel they can ask questions that they perceive as challenging without offending their clinician.[19]

A second study on patient perceptions of safety in the hospital found that practices that we may consider routine in the healthcare setting are new to the patient.[20] However, it turns out that if we engage the patient in even a brief interaction—asking the patient to say her name out loud while the nurse reads the name on the label, for example—it can return an important sense of control to the patient.

That's what happens when we choose to sit instead of stand. When we ignore the impulse to save time by standing at the end of the patient's bed or at the door to the exam room in favor of sitting down, we open the door to conversation. In fact, studies even show that patients tend to overestimate the amount of time a physician spent with them when they sit. They also report a more positive interaction and a better understanding of their condition.[21]

Celebrate Progress Together

It sounds so simple, doesn't it? But too often, in the interest of quickly meeting the needs of the next patient, physicians and other caregivers miss a wonderful opportunity to connect back to their desire for purposeful, worthwhile work that makes a difference for the patient they're with. It's so important because that's what provides momentum for *their* engagement.

Many of our patients are on a marathon journey to shift their health. They may take years to make meaningful change. But nobody makes it to the finish line without lots of encouragement along the way. Patients need it and so do those who care for them.

Clinicians who do it best find small wins to celebrate. While a patient may not yet meet his goal of controlling his hemoglobin A1C down to a level of seven or less, he may well be controlling it better than he was last time his physician saw him. So celebrate that.

Likewise, that overweight patient may not have yet lost the 30 pounds she's aiming for, but she did lose those first three pounds. Cheer her on. Ask her what she did differently over the last month to achieve that. Express confidence that she's building good habits for even greater success. Celebrate progress together because it fuels everyone's engagement.

Engaging Special Patient Populations

No discussion of how to effectively engage patients would be complete without recognizing the importance of adapting your engagement approach to different groups of patients with distinct needs. The goal is to always be sensitive to the unique needs of the patient at hand so you can appropriately address any barriers to a positive patient experience and quality clinical outcomes.

While it's beyond the scope of this book to delve into the unique attributes of the many special patient populations that clinicians see, let's consider at least a few of the most common:

Patients with ethnic, racial, and gender differences—It's easy to minimize the influence of race and ethnicity in healthcare today or confuse it with socioeconomic status. As one author of a healthcare blog explains, we assume that "people like us" share our communication preferences, for one thing.[22] But here's the reality: While patients from different racial and ethnic groups share similar expectations of their physicians, they report different types of experiences.[23]

One study reported, for instance, that "Physicians were more contentious with black patients whom they perceived as less effective communicators and less satisfied."[24] Another author examining the influence of race and ethnicity on patient activation concluded that "Blacks and Hispanics generally perceive their role relationships with physicians to be less equitable than do whites."[25]

The same study also suggested that for Hispanics, activation was possibly affected more by characteristics like compassion, care, and sensitivity to language. In fact, that's been the experience of Columbia Valley Community Health (CVCH), a federally qualified health center in Wenatchee, WA, with a large Hispanic population.

At CVCH, 40 percent of patients speak Spanish and tend to exhibit cultural characteristics—like being respectful but passive when they don't understand—that can cause misunderstandings with clinicians. As a result, all clinicians at CVCH are fluent in Spanish. In fact, if they're not, they attend a three-week immersion program in Guatemala. Even still, translators are available to help with complex or nuanced communications.

In addition, clinicians use motivational interviewing techniques to ensure patients hear what they are saying. "It's a two-directional communication approach," explains CEO Patrick Bucknum. "They begin by assessing whether a patient is ready to hear what they are going to say and also use the teach-back method at the end to ensure key points were understood and to assess a patient's willingness to follow the physician's advice."[26]

CVCH is so committed to hardwiring its patient perspective in everything it does that its Board of Directors actually mirrors its patient population, including Spanish-only speakers and a migrant farm worker. "They tell us about the issues patients are trying to communicate that we aren't hearing," adds Bucknum.

"Whether it's that a clinic or department name doesn't translate well to Spanish or the fact that we need another adult dentist, they bring what the survey responses are trying to tell us into the boardroom. They use that frontline perspective to shape a more meaningful strategic plan."[27]

There are gender differences to consider when engaging patients, too. For example, some have postulated that women are more likely than men to take medication as prescribed when they perceive a collaborative relationship with their physician. Also, women are more likely to be health information seekers than men are.[28]

Disadvantaged patients—Sometimes socioeconomic and racial disparities in health combine to reduce access to care. One clinical trial that launched in August 2016 is examining the impact of patient engagement on improving experience and care for this population.[29]

The study, which includes 360 African Americans and Latinos with knee osteoarthritis, plans to roll out to eight sites across the U.S. and examine the impact of a shared decision-making tool for better outcomes. The problem is that this group underutilizes knee replacements, and when they do opt for them, they have higher rates of adverse outcomes.

The study hypothesizes that this is likely due to a complex mix of factors, such as living in poverty or a food desert, lack of information, and fear about undergoing treatment that keeps such patients living in pain when they could be fully functional.

The hope is that when patients in this study who have been content to do nothing can compare wearing a brace or getting a knee replacement with delaying or forgoing treatment, they will better appreciate the cost of doing nothing and make more informed choices.

Health disparities—like drug and chemical dependency or mental health disorders—often trigger poverty or symptoms of poverty that complicate the patient's ability to understand and act upon the very treatment options that would make a meaningful difference. Sometimes the barriers are more practical in nature, like lack of transportation or money to fill a prescription.

> ## Sometimes the barriers are more practical in nature, like lack of transportation or money to fill a prescription.

Because patients at CVCH typically struggle with these issues, the organization has honed its ability to break down barriers whenever it finds them. One of the sources of anxiety that they uncovered for patients was sitting on an exam table.[30]

Since just one in five patients needs to disrobe for an exam, CVCH replaced two out of three of each clinician's exam rooms with "talking rooms." The new rooms facilitate patient-clinician conversation without raising anxiety and blood pressure, as is common for patients who sit on an exam table.

An Engaged Clinician Makes All the Difference

As I walked into the exam room to meet my patient, Trish, I glanced at the intake form, which said she was a "43-year-old female with fatigue." I looked up and noted that she was sitting hunched forward, head in her hands, looking defeated.

I introduced myself, sat down, and invited her to share her story. Addicted to drugs and caught dealing, Trish had been in prison for the last few years. During her final months, she transitioned to a work crew, but struggled to keep up due to her worsening fatigue.

"I'm tired all the time. I can't lift the trash bags or the tools. I just want to sit down and rest," she explained. Trish told me she had a heart murmur and was told to follow up a few years ago, but never did. She told me about her drug addiction and contracting hepatitis C from dirty needles. She shared about her 10-year sobriety and the devastating relapse that sent her back to prison and her two teenage kids to live with their grandparents.

And she shared her experiences in healthcare: the condescending looks when a clinician or staff person read "history of drug abuse" in her chart…the instantaneous judgment she felt and the flippant dismissals she received, as if she were worthless, not worthy of their time.

That was until she came to Columbia Valley Community Health. She told me that the people at CVCH treat her differently. They show her respect. They look her in the eye. They listen to her. They treat her like a person, not an addict. She feels safe and at home here. She comes in to share the joy of her ongoing sobriety. And she comes in to sit and cry when the pressures of life just seem too much.

At that first visit, I listened to her heart and heard a very worrisome murmur. We immediately sent her for further imaging and on to cardiac surgery. Within two weeks, she was back in my office with a new heart valve that likely saved her life.

Throughout the stress of an urgent heart surgery, Trish often called our care coordination nurse, Brigette, or messaged her through the portal. Brigette talked her through the various tests, calmed her fears about the upcoming surgery, coordinated numerous appointments, and above all, *listened* to Trish.

As a team, we made sure Trish didn't fall through the cracks again. There are good days and bad days for Trish. She still suffers from severe depression, a broken family, and the mistakes of her past. But now, she has a place to come for support, help, and a listening ear. The last vestiges of her life as an addict are slowly falling away, and they reveal the valuable human being that is Trish.

—Allie Ivanowicz, PA-C
Columbia Valley Community Health
Wenatchee, WA

Patients with generational differences—For the first time ever, there are four generations together in the workplace: traditionalists, baby boomers, Generation Xers, and millennials. It's important to understand that our experiences during our formative years help define us and shape how we view the world.

So it's perhaps no surprise that there are some very real differences between the preferences of millennials and Gen X patients and their parents and grandparents when they access and consume healthcare. For instance, many members of the greatest generation and some baby boomers don't feel comfortable using certain technologies and would prefer a physician to take more time with them over the convenience of a quick appointment.[31]

We risk disengaging those individuals if we force text message appointment reminders and emails upon them. But it's a catch-22 since technology can also help this population—who will become heavy consumers of healthcare in the near-term as they enter their golden years—to do more for themselves at home.[32]

In contrast, millennials and Gen Xers, who have grown up with social media, YouTube, and Google, have a very different set of needs and desires. While they expect quality care, they also prefer convenience and quick appointments. This group is enthusiastic, adaptable, inclusive, and self-sufficient.

They want to be heard and asked for their input. Some studies show that they also tend to have a lower sense of commitment and a tendency toward more of a "know-it-all" attitude than their parents do. It's important to them that you communicate the meaning and purpose of your organization.[33]

The organizations that will be most effective at engaging patients in the years to come will find creative ways to understand, assess, accept, and respond to the very different communication needs among each of these generations.

Patients with different levels of activation—So far, we've considered special populations in general terms—i.e., racial or generational differences—but the most meaningful measure we can use, by far, will be differentiating our engagement approach based on an *individual* patient's actual activation.

> **The most meaningful measure we can use, by far, will be differentiating our engagement approach based on an *individual* patient's actual activation.**

There's some exciting applications of Dr. Hibbard's research with Patient Activation Measures (PAM) already occurring in healthcare today...ways in which organizations are sorting actual patients to better engage them. A number of organizations are tracking PAM and tailoring customized care pathways based on the level of activation.

For example, an innovative Stanford clinic that sees Stanford University employees and their family members with expensive, serious health challenges uses PAM to determine which patients need more support (i.e., low scorers) from specially trained medical assistants. As a result, Stanford can identify the most efficient way to spend its resources to meet patient needs.[34]

A health insurer has used PAM scores in a similar way recently to segment support in three areas—physician support, emotional support, and navigational support—for patients with a cancer diagnosis. High scorers—activated patients—get access to a menu of web-based resources while low scorers get a live coach. The results? Higher patient satisfaction across the board while reducing costs by half.[35]

Another organization uses PAM scores to tailor care pathways for patients with back pain by pairing a pain acuity score with the PAM so that high scorers on both measures might visit a physical therapist once a week to learn exercises while low scorers might visit three times per week for more support.[36]

If we want to engage patients in meaningful ways, we will need to demonstrate our nuanced understanding of what matters to patients through a comprehensive strategy that, once again, *meets patients where they are*, and systematically deconstructs barriers to a truly patient-centered agenda. It's an exciting time in healthcare today.

Patient Engagement: What Wrong Looks Like

When Donna got a notice in the mail that she was due for her annual mammogram as well as a colonoscopy, she rolled her eyes and promptly threw it in the trash. Despite seeing the same primary care physician for the last decade, he hadn't inspired her to keep current with her annual well woman exam.

The last time she'd seen him, he stood across the room with his hand practically on the doorknob as he ran through a quick list of questions. He seemed frazzled when he mentioned he was going to add a new medication so Donna just nodded. She knew she'd never fill it because it was expensive and she usually forgot to take her medicines anyway.

Plus, she never heard back from anyone at the clinic after she did a recommended lab or test. They simply looked over her chart on the next visit and said it had been "completed." What was the point of getting a $300 bill from insurance for "completed"?

Nope, she decided, the mammogram she did 10 years ago and the colonoscopy she did 20 years ago were good enough for her. They'd been "completed."

Patient Engagement: What Right Looks Like

When Donna answered the phone, it was her doctor's office reminding her that her appointment for her annual well woman visit was scheduled for next Monday, July 14, at 2 p.m. "Dr. Kayson asked me to tell you he's looking forward to seeing you," she said. "So I just wanted to take a quick moment to see if you needed directions and go over your co-pay that will be due when you arrive."

Donna had been thinking about skipping out on the appointment, but since Dr. Kayson seemed to be expecting her, she confirmed it instead. When she arrived for her appointment, she was greeted by the front desk clerk who, upon hearing her name, said: "Dr. Kayson is looking forward to seeing you this morning. He's running on time and we should be able to get you back there in about 10 minutes. Thanks for being early!"

When Dr. Kayson arrived for her exam, she noticed that he immediately pulled up his chair close to hers and gave her his full attention. So she returned the courtesy. Then he asked her what was most important to her in her visit that day.

She explained that she just wasn't sure about the whole mammogram and colonoscopy thing because there might be out-of-pocket expenses her insurance wouldn't cover and money was tight right now. Plus, she was busy with the kids so she didn't know when she'd actually get around to making an appointment.

Dr. Kayson explained that she was overdue for her last mammogram and explained the American Cancer Society's recommendation that women her age should be screened annually and why. He also shared a bit about why he felt colonoscopies could be such a life-saving screening tool for colon cancer when patients followed through with consistent screenings.

By the time he told Donna that his assistant could schedule the two appointments for her, she was all in. Because Dr. Kayson concluded the visit by saying, "I've just shared a lot of information with you. What questions may

I answer?" Donna was able to ask when she'd receive the results of the screenings and knew when to follow up in case she didn't hear anything.

When Dr. Kayson's nurse called a week later to follow up from her appointment, she shared the good news that both screenings were negative.

Those procedures were worth every penny for peace of mind, Donna reflected. And Dr. Kayson was a real find.

Key Learning Points: Engaging Patients and Families

1. Physicians and other clinicians can most impact patient engagement by building trust through expertise and empathy, individualizing the care, empowering and partnering with patients, and celebrating progress together.

2. Six Studer Group tools respond directly to these drivers of patient engagement: AIDET, Individualized Patient Care, Bedside Shift Report, Hourly Rounding, nurse leader rounding, and pre- and post-visit phone calls.

3. When clinicians sit (versus stand) with patients, it flattens the authority gradient so that patients are comfortable, don't feel rushed, and are more likely to ask questions and share information.

4. An engagement strategy for patients from special populations deserves special consideration. These populations include patients with ethnic, racial, and gender differences; disadvantaged patients; and generational differences. Sorting patients by actual activation level through PAM scores is a promising new trend.

PART FOUR

Processes and Tools That Support
Patient Engagement

While clinicians can have a significant impact on patient engagement, those opportunities are brief. As we've discussed, the average patient sees a doctor just 20 minutes three times per year. Every moment must count since it will influence the patient's choices in the many thousands of remaining hours when the patient is not in the physician's office.

Many would argue that this lack of face time is one of the greatest challenges in improving health outcomes and lowering costs. In fact, recently I heard just this complaint from a retired physician after my presentation to the medical staff at a large teaching hospital during a Grand Rounds session. He told me that he felt this lack of time between him and his patients was why he left medicine. He explained that many of his patients needed two, three, or even more hours with him at least monthly to make significant progress in improving their health.

He explained that he'd practiced medicine in that community for more than 40 years and had seen changes in healthcare that I'd only read about in texts. He was just so frustrated by the continuing pressures to see more patients in less time. So we talked for a while about what could be done.

We agreed that market forces shaping how we get paid for patient visits wasn't likely to add more money for seeing these patients any time soon. But as we talked through the problem, we also agreed that not every patient needed more time. After all, as I pointed out, while I'd thoroughly enjoy longer visits with my own doctor, the reality is that, as a healthy individual, more care probably isn't better care. In fact, the opposite is often true.

However, we're fortunate to live in an age where there are dozens of new resources that weren't available in the past to support clinicians and fill in some of those interstitial spaces. The best of them do just that—they aim to support rather than replace clinicians. But they can't do it alone. To success-fully engage patients, we need to embrace creative ways of redesigning our organizations to put consumers squarely at the center of their care...so it's easy and intuitive for them to get the care they need.

Let's look next at some solutions that hold the most promise for both serving as an extension of the caregiver and making a meaningful difference in a patient's ability to take charge of his own health.

CHAPTER 7

Beyond the Caregiver—The Role of Technology and Organizational Design in Patient Engagement

Earlier, I shared a bit about the push within the health industry to embrace patient portals as an engagement strategy. While they are insufficient as a standalone strategy, they *do* offer vast potential to engage patients when used in conjunction with many of the other tools and tactics we've reviewed thus far.

In fact, one study examined the value of IT platforms in patient engagement in a systematic review of 170 articles on the topic and found that their use does indeed correlate with better health outcomes and engaged patient behaviors, although more research needs to be done to standardize the ways in which this is measured.[1] To be effective, the use of patient portals needs to be fine-tuned to engage the patients who need it most.

Do We Collect the *Right* Information about Patients?

Remember our discussion about Target and its ability to predict which customers are pregnant in order to send them coupons for diapers and other baby-related items to preempt competitors? That's an important difference between the data we collect in electronic health records and the capabilities of engagement experts in other consumer-focused industries. They don't just collect the data; they actually *use* it to get better results.

What would you do in your organization if you had access to the predictive analytics and team of behavioral economists who sift through and apply

Target's data? Would you pre-call no-shows or patients who typically arrive late like Warner Thomas at Ochsner recommended?

That's essentially the definition of precision medicine: the ability to respond to the unique needs of individual patients. The National Institutes of Health says it is: "disease treatment and prevention that takes into account individual variability in genes, environment, and lifestyle for each person." But what if we took that idea a step further to collect and respond to *all* the unique attributes that make each person the individual that they are?

A simple physical exam neglects so much key information. For instance, we can understand the whole person only if we also take into account his motivations, influences, personal health goals, and family. Psychosocial assessments, which are often overlooked during physical exams, can be particularly useful here.

What should be included in such an assessment? I like the acronym "SELF PACING" as a way to remember what information to collect during a comprehensive exam:

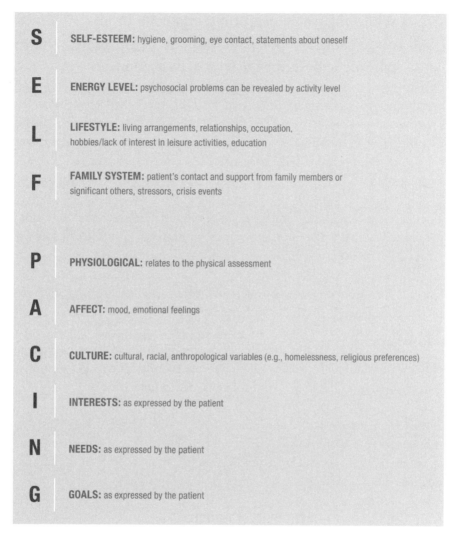

S   **SELF-ESTEEM:** hygiene, grooming, eye contact, statements about oneself

E   **ENERGY LEVEL:** psychosocial problems can be revealed by activity level

L   **LIFESTYLE:** living arrangements, relationships, occupation, hobbies/lack of interest in leisure activities, education

F   **FAMILY SYSTEM:** patient's contact and support from family members or significant others, stressors, crisis events

P   **PHYSIOLOGICAL:** relates to the physical assessment

A   **AFFECT:** mood, emotional feelings

C   **CULTURE:** cultural, racial, anthropological variables (e.g., homelessness, religious preferences)

I   **INTERESTS:** as expressed by the patient

N   **NEEDS:** as expressed by the patient

G   **GOALS:** as expressed by the patient

Figure 7.1 | SELF PACING

Source: ArcMesa Educators. "Psychosocial Assessment." *Nursing Link,* http://nursinglink.monster.com/training/articles/296-physical-assessment---chapter-10-psychosocial-assessment.

Neglecting to collect so much key information at the outset is a real challenge when it comes to engaging patients effectively. While electronic health records contain lots of clinical and financial information about our patients, there's nothing to describe the patient as a *person.*

While electronic health records contain lots of clinical and financial information about our patients, there's nothing to describe the patient as a *person*.

We also need to understand the barriers to engagement. Did a patient neglect to show up because she lives in the city and takes the bus, but we referred her to a specialist in the suburbs? A referral to a specialist who can be accessed via public transportation will dramatically increase the chances the appointment is kept.

These are the same kinds of lifestyle issues that determine whether or not a patient will actually fill a prescription at the pharmacy. One CEO I spoke to recently told me this was his biggest learning of the year.

He said that a number of his leaders had spent time shadowing caregivers in the emergency department to better understand their organization and were stunned to hear about the many challenges patients had in filling their prescriptions. Because they didn't have an on-site discharge pharmacy where patients could fill prescriptions before leaving, they decided to add a question during discharge: "How will your fill your medications today?"

If the patient answered that they didn't know or didn't have a clear plan, then they began to look for ways to fill them before the patient left or to deliver them directly at home. Understanding such a basic barrier to obtaining a quality clinical outcome is just so critical.

Give Clinicians Actionable Information

Another barrier to filling medications or following up on a physician referral that is frequently underappreciated is health literacy. In this case, we're not just talking about "functional literacy," reading well enough to conduct oneself and hold a job or read a bus map, for example. Health literacy requires another set of skills. We need to ensure that a patient can obtain, process, and understand enough health information to be informed and engaged.

In one PAM study, Dr. Hibbard noted that 25 percent of health literacy is predicted by socio-economic variables while those same socio-economic variables predict just 5 to 6 percent of the PAM score. In other words, it's very difficult to look at an individual and—based on a person's income, ethnicity, and years of college—determine whether they are engaged.

> **In one PAM study, Dr. Hibbard noted that 25 percent of health literacy is predicted by socio-economic variables while those same socio-economic variables predict just 5 to 6 percent of the PAM score.**

The American Medical Association offers a training video on health literacy for physicians to sensitize them to these issues. You can watch an abbreviated four-minute version with patient vignettes on YouTube that might surprise you.[2] In the video, one physician interviews a college office assistant who entered a literacy program at a seventh grade reading level. She explains that she was sick a lot because she didn't take her medicines as prescribed since she couldn't read and didn't want anyone to know. So she didn't ask questions of her doctor.

In another vignette, a respected church deacon who reads at the third grade level is reading the instructions aloud to his physician as she has requested. He says, "one capsule twice daily." His physician nods and says, "So how would you take it?" "Well," he says, "it says twice daily but it doesn't say what time to take it."

A third patient who reads at a fifth grade level talks about the stress of needing to fill out a form as soon as he arrives at a doctor's visit…how it makes his heart race and he's tempted to turn around and walk out…because he can't read well enough to complete that form. If we expect patients to fully participate in owning their healthcare, it's got to be non-negotiable to understand their level of health literacy. Only then can we respond in ways that reduce anxiety and build the trust that forms the foundation for patient engagement.

Thinking beyond the basics—like psychosocial assessments and health literacy—what about PAM scores? In Chapter 6, I shared with you how a health insurer is using PAM scores to sort cancer patients so that activated patients have access to web-based resources while low scorers get a live coach.

Just imagine the power of knowing a patient's actual level of activation and capturing it in the patient's electronic health record for a clinician to use in designing a treatment plan during that patient's visit. What a powerful determinant of a quality clinical outcome it would be. In fact, it's tools like these that will move us from the *idea* of population health to the *reality* of precision medicine in the years to come.

Technology Must Help, Not Hinder

My Studer Group® colleague, Dr. Gurpreet Dhaliwal, who is a professor of clinical medicine at the University of California San Francisco, and arguably one of the most brilliant diagnosticians in healthcare today, is quick to confirm that technology is not a patient engagement strategy. It's a *tool* that can be helpful when it supports a physician's ability to engage a patient.

He says it's critical that caregivers *invite the patient into the conversation.* Just consider the power of a physician's response to a patient who explains that she's been recording her blood sugar multiple times a day over many weeks. If the physician says, "Thank you for doing this. It's helpful," it opens the door to engagement.

But if the physician says, "We don't use blood sugars anymore. We use the A1C test instead," it's very dismissive. The patient shuts down. Patients may worry that their input is trivial or they sound uninformed, when, actually, that input is the safety check we require.

Dr. Dhaliwal is concerned about the instances where technology is a distraction from the patient engagement we are trying to foster, such as when a patient with diabetes is spending so much time monitoring his glucose that he neglects other critical components of his care, like his diet and exercise. In fact, it turns out that willpower is a finite, but "replenishable" resource...

something that's important to appreciate as you try to engage patients in building healthy new habits.

In one study, researchers divided college students into two groups. They placed a plate of freshly baked chocolate chip cookies in front of both groups, but allowed only one group to eat them. The other group had to eat radishes instead. Then, they compared the performance of the two groups on completing a puzzle, a task to gauge perseverance, used as a proxy for willpower here.

The surprising results? It was the cookie eaters who performed better...not the radish eaters. That's because the radish eaters had already "spent" some of their willpower reserves in resisting the cookies, while the cookie eaters had not. They therefore had less willpower to draw on and puzzle performance suffered.[3]

In the spirit of inviting patients into the conversation, Dr. Dhaliwal might say to a diabetes patient who is over-monitoring at the expense of other healthy behaviors, "It would be OK if you cut down your measuring and recording time and spend the time that you would've been monitoring on taking a daily walk instead."

At Studer Group's 2016 What's Right in Health Care® Conference, Dr. Dhaliwal gave a fascinating talk about whether he believes robots will replace doctors someday. He says that, while he is a big advocate of artificial intelligence and the value of learning from machines, computers won't replace doctors. He believes that computers someday may excel at knowing what's the matter with a patient, but they will never know what matters *to* a patient.

Do we understand what the patient's personal health goals are? Not the goals "prescribed" by the physician...but the quality of life that the patient ultimately desires. Just think back to the story I shared earlier about the patient who was disengaged because she'd expressed a desire for fruit daily in the hospital. When she overheard employees making disparaging remarks about her request in the hallway, it negatively affected her whole hospital experience. How could a computer understand that?

Diagnosis requires understanding medicine and understanding people. A computer has to be programmed to know a patient doesn't want to be in pain. It would also have to be programmed to understand the full range of human emotions. Since such programming isn't realistic, its ability to diagnose in a way that solves the real-life problem a human being is facing from their illness is very limited indeed.

Also, Dr. Dhaliwal notes, the best diagnosticians in the world share something in common: the sheer joy of diagnosis…something a computer just can't replicate. (Just ponder for a moment Click and Clack, the Tappet brothers, on NPR's award-winning radio show *Car Talk*. Not only do they exemplify the qualities of good diagnosticians, but if you've ever "wasted another perfectly good hour listening to the show," you understand how that kind of joy is contagious and could never be replicated by a machine.)

And yet, technology can be incredibly useful if we use it in novel ways to support the caregiver in doing what matters most to him: delivering quality clinical care and a positive patient experience. When it comes to electronic health records, he laments—like most physicians today—the fact that we've added in so much information to the record that the act of moving through it for a physician is no longer about the patient. From quality and safety to drug ordering and entering diets, it's one big black hole that detracts from time in the patient encounter.

Sadly, while technology in every area of our lives has made things faster and more efficient, no one would ever claim that about the EHR. The thing is: The EHR has dozens of stakeholders (i.e., the lawyers, the insurers, the hospitals) but it has just one data entry clerk…and that person is called the *physician*.

Dr. Dhaliwal fantasizes about a future where physicians would get some return for all the typing they do…a sort of "assist" in the job they do to make them smarter. For instance, if the EHR was intelligent, when the doctor typed in "heartburn" for a diagnosis, a note might pop up that: "Doctors who like heartburn also like heart attack"…just as Amazon suggests to readers of books on cars that they might like related titles about books on motorcycles.

While this kind of artificial intelligence is still a long way away (in medicine, anyway), it's probably coming. Already, the computer will alert a physician entering a prescription about a dangerous interaction with another drug the patient is taking. In an ideal world, however, the kind of technology Dr. Dhaliwal is hoping for is nuanced…it feels more like a valued colleague offering a second opinion. While we're not there yet, there are some excellent examples of what's already making a meaningful difference in the lives of patients.

When Technology Boosts Engagement

We need look no further than healthcare's younger generation of physicians to understand the promise of technology in patient engagement today. Here's why: They are using handheld ultrasounds just as often as older doctors used stethoscopes.

In a short exam that doesn't always allow for ample interaction with a busy doctor, this sends a clear message to patients: "I want to be accurate so I am using the best technology." It also offers a way to connect with the patient in an age when physicians have to work hard to not seem *dis*engaged as they type mountains of information into the EHR. Handheld ultrasounds are a great example of technology that meets the physician's diagnostic needs while *improving* engagement.

Another example: Have you heard of the insanely popular Pokémon GO game? It's the mobile app that's driving millennials (and some of their parents) to obsessively "collect" Pokémon creatures in real-world locations through a cell phone's GPS and camera. At one Michigan children's hospital, creative caregivers are using the app to get kids out of bed and moving around as they chase Pokémons around the hospital.[4] They've even noted that patients will stop and help each other pose for a picture with a Pokémon they can see only on their phone. Talk about engagement!

Some healthcare organizations are responding enthusiastically to patient interest in cell phone apps like these. At Studer Group's What's Right in Health Care conference, Ochsner CEO Warner Thomas also talked about his organization's commitment to culling through the best technology has to offer and enlisting it in their effort to engage patients. In fact, they invite patients to belly up to the organization's very own "O" bar to get set up with apps to control their diseases.

Recently, Ochsner enrolled 700 patients with hypertension in a trial using Apple Watches to remind them to move more and take their medications on time. Patients loved it. Not only that, but while the average number of patients who are typically able to control blood pressure within six months of treatment is 13 percent, fully 60 percent of the Apple Watch wearers achieved that during Ochsner's trial.

Even Aetna is getting in on the action. In fall 2016, it announced it would make the Apple Watch available to certain large employers and individual customers during open enrollment, becoming the first major healthcare company to actually subsidize a portion of the cost. The company even provides Apple Watches to its nearly 50,000 employees at no cost.[5]

Wearable devices like these have exploded recently, with 245 million devices projected for sale by 2019.[6] And healthcare providers are getting on board. For example, Dana-Farber Cancer Institute has launched a new study partnering with Fitbit to manage obesity in women with early breast cancer. Also, at the Nebraska College of Medicine, a neuroscientist has launched a device that looks like a watch to track tremors for Parkinson's patients. The data is collected in a mobile app that then facilitates discussion—a great way to invite the patient in—during office visits.[7]

Sometimes, though, it's the simple things that can make the difference when it comes to technology. Like email reminders to patients. This is important when you consider that between 40 and 80 percent of what a caregiver tells patients is quickly forgotten, and half of what they do remember, they get wrong.[8]

> **Sometimes, though, it's the simple things that can make the difference when it comes to technology. Like email reminders to patients.**

In a UCLA trial, researchers set out to see if they could improve those numbers by sharing their physician's notes—using a program called OpenNotes—directly with patients and sending them email reminders to log on and review those notes. Researchers hailed the trial as an unqualified success. Patients demonstrated better recall of their medical plans, felt a stronger sense of control in their care, and took their medications more reliably.[9]

An interesting side note about these findings: While doctors were initially concerned that the email reminders would cause excess patient emails and interfere with their workflow, it turned out to be a non-issue. When doctors were offered the opportunity to opt out, none of them did.

The power of these emails became even more compelling when Geisinger Health System, due to an electronic glitch, stopped providing the email reminders to view OpenNotes after providing them for a year. Researchers found that while 60.9 percent of Geisinger patients checked their doctor's notes during the first year, just 13.2 percent did in year two after the email reminders were interrupted.[10]

Remember our earlier discussion about the need to step up outreach to engage special populations? The data in this study confirmed that. It noted less viewership by patients from disadvantaged backgrounds and/or lower health literacy, and recommended a more proactive approach to engaging those patients.

As you begin to consider ways to integrate technology for higher engagement into your own organization, it can be useful to consider a phased approach that builds on the natural stages of engagement. For instance, the Healthcare Information and Management Systems Society Foundation (HIMSS) has developed a five-stage model of patient engagement framework that suggests tools and tactics that become progressively more sophisticated. Each stage aligns with the various stages of meaningful use as well.

Patient Engagement Framework

Inform Me	Engage Me	Empower Me	Partner With Me	Support My e-Community
Information and Way-Finding	Information and Way-Finding	Information, Way-Finding, and Quality	Information, Way-Finding, and Analytics/Quality	Information, Way-Finding, and Analytics/Quality
e-Tools	e-Tools	e-Tools	e-Tools	e-Visits and e-Tools
Forms: Printable	Interactive Forms: Online	Integrated Forms: EHR	Integrated Forms: EHR	Integrated Forms: EHR
Patient-Specific Education	Patient-Specific Education	Patient-Specific Education	Patient-Specific Education	Patient-Specific Education
	Patient Access: Records	Patient Access: Records	Patient Access	Patient Access and Use
		Patient-Generated Data	Patient-Generated Data	Care Team-Generated Data
		Interoperable Records	Interoperable Records	Interoperable Records
			Collaborative Care	Collaborative Care
				Community Support
Aligned: Emerging Meaningful Use	**Aligned:** Meaningful Use 1	**Aligned:** Meaningful Use 2	**Aligned:** Meaningful Use 3	**Aligned:** Meaningful Use 4+

Figure 7.2 | Simplified HIMSS Patient Engagement Framework

As you can see in the graphic above, the HIMSS framework begins with a simplified patient-centric approach, offering information and "way-finding" tools, e-tools, printable forms, and patient-specific education to inform and impact patients. This approach then builds with more resources to "retain and interact," then to "partner effectively," and finally to "create synergy and extend reach."

Because we've omitted a great deal of useful detail for the purposes of illustration here, I recommend you view and download HIMSS's complete framework at http://www.himss.org/himss-patient-engagement-framework. Then you'll see how the sophistication in engaging patients increases dramatically at each of these five phases.

For example, while "information and way finding" resources in the "Inform Me" stage might include maps and directions and a physician directory, in the "Partner with Me" stage, it also includes analytics and quality indicators with things like patient-specific quality indicators and patient accountability scores. By the time patients are engaged in a true e-community, they are able to compare costs, quality, and convenience for providers, treatments, and medications. See HIMSS's original graphic for complete details.

E-Health Is Coming Quickly

No discussion about the use of technology in patient engagement would be complete with mentioning the rapid pace by which consumers are adopting telehealth. There are a number of reasons that the trend is taking off. First, it's delivering results and saving patients money. Secondly, satisfaction with telehealth is very high. And third, consumers are demanding more convenient access to high-quality care (as we see with the proliferation of CVS-style clinics as discussed earlier).

In short, telehealth delivers on each of these fronts. Another contributor to the speed of this growing trend is the Centers for Medicare & Medicaid Services, which has announced that its next generation ACO model will cover telehealth beyond what's currently allowable.

Telehealth—which encompasses a variety of technologies to deliver virtual medical service—has been enthusiastically embraced by American consumers. In 2015, there were approximately 800,000 online consultations in the U.S. with an anticipated increase to 7 million in 2018.[11] That's pretty dramatic growth, particularly when you compare it to the 350,000 visits just a few years earlier.[12]

It's perhaps not surprising that consumers are embracing telehealth so readily. In fact, I've used it several times myself—as well as for one of my sons—and had great experiences. Of the four times I used the service (each time for upper respiratory issues), I was prescribed antibiotics just twice.

In the other instances, I instead received the peace of mind that comes from a physician reassuring me that the symptoms pointed toward a viral infection and that there would be no need for a prescription. As someone interested in quality and safety, this won me over.

The current leader of telehealth is a company called Teladoc, which is larger than all three of its top competitors combined. In fact, Teladoc owns over 70 percent of the telehealth market, with a network of over 2,900 MD-credentialed behavioral health and dermatology professionals.[13]

67% of healthcare professionals either use some form of telemedicine now or are planning to in the next 3 years

>70% of consumers would rather have an online video visit to obtain a prescription than travel to their doctor's office

91% of health outcomes were as good or better via telehealth

63.5% of patients would be comfortable conducting a virtual appointment at home

Figure 7.3 | Consumers are enthusiastic about telehealth.
Source: Hyatt, Ali. "Top 10 Stats to Know About Telehealth," *Webside Matters* (blog), American Well, January 21, 2015, https://www.americanwell.com/top-10-stats-you-need-to-know-about-telehealth/.

We're Getting Technology Backward

Despite the tremendous advances that healthcare apps and telehealth are already delivering to patients, we still risk getting technology backward. Just as we discussed with respect to patient portals, technology is most useful once you have an engaged patient. It can't *make* patients become engaged. And sometimes—as is the case with patient portals—we may be missing the patients we need to engage most…those who aren't interested or skilled with technology.

What we *can* do is focus first on using technology to remove old-fashioned barriers to engagement. Why, for example, does healthcare have such a fragmented system of patient records? We frequently expect patients to show up to a doctor's appointment with a paper copy of a test result in hand since we may not have it.

There are no insurmountable technological reasons why a patient's electronic health record doesn't share information with each of a patient's healthcare providers. There's also not a good reason why medical devices don't share data...or why hospital pricing is not transparent or easy to understand.[14] Maybe when we think about how we can use technology to engage patients, we should start there. Because really, is it the patient's responsibility—or our own responsibility—to transform a broken system?

Designing a Patient-Centric Organization

When we think about how to design a better organization that puts patient interests first, let's begin by ensuring that we always capture the voice of the customer, not just for honing our marketing messages, but for genuinely improving our tools and processes to be more patient-friendly. For example, consider the common challenge of timely lab results. Late and missing lab results contribute to legions of errors, especially pernicious delays in diagnosis when a significant result isn't acted upon quickly enough.

There's a simple way to get deeper insights on this: The Agency for Healthcare Research and Quality (AHRQ) has developed a patient engagement survey to assess patients' understanding of tests and knowledge about what to do after receiving their test results.[15]

It's a common problem. Patients don't understand why a test was ordered or when to expect results. Or, they assume that "no news is good news" and so don't take the initiative to get their results when they are late. A quick patient survey can change all that by asking patients directly if they understand tests that have been ordered, when to expect results, what to do if they don't hear about results when they are due, and how they prefer to be contacted.

The survey can be administered either after a patient has ordered/completed a test (but before the results are back) or after a patient has been notified of their test results. An optional question can be used for offices where patient follow-up is a problem.

But let's consider the common, larger healthcare experience for a moment from the patient perspective. If you were a new patient in a primary care practice at a major academic medical center, you'd likely be re-routed through two or three automated phone trees before you were fortunate enough to finally get an appointment three weeks into the future.

Is that the first impression we want to make? It's particularly concerning because from a patient perspective, there's this huge disparity between the challenge of consuming healthcare and everything else in their lives. Think about the Apple iPhone. If you want to listen to a Bob Dylan tune, you simply press a button, put in your ear buds, relax, and enjoy. Even though it's an enormous feat of engineering to make that happen so seamlessly for you, the complexity is hidden.

Now think about the last hospital bill you or a loved one received. Or rather, think about the flurry of hospital bills that you received. You likely received one bill from the emergency department and many others from the medical practices of the various specialists you saw.

And then, when you thought you'd paid all the bills, a big bill from the hospital itself arrived in the mailbox. But wait...that's the cost *before* your insurance had paid its portion, so you are not really supposed to pay it. Are you kidding me?

The whole process is completely bewildering to the average consumer, much less those of us who actually work in the industry. Of course, there are hundreds of examples like these in healthcare today...where we expect the patient to navigate incredible complexity to receive care, at a time when he may be feeling worried, anxious, and ill.

Some medical specialties are making inroads, though. Management of cancer, for example, is a 24-hour job between the appointments, medications, radiation therapy, and diet management. Because leaving the coordination of such complex care in the hands of a sick patient and his family makes no sense, some organizations that care for these patients make nurse navigators available to patients.

The concept of patient navigation began in 1990 with Dr. Harold Freeman, a surgical oncologist at Harlem Hospital in New York. Dr. Freeman was interested in eliminating barriers to cancer screening, diagnosis, treatment, and care for underserved and minority patients in the area.[16]

Because many of Harlem's patients were impoverished and half had no medical insurance on the initial visit, fully 49 percent of breast cancer patients presented with stage 3 and 4 disease before the nurse navigator intervention. The five-year survival rate was 39 percent. But after early intervention with free and low-cost exams and access to nurse navigators, the survival rate jumped to 70 percent.[17]

Ultimately, in 2005—and in large part due to these very results at Harlem Hospital—Congress passed an act that ultimately resulted in funding for the National Institutes of Health's Center to Reduce Cancer Disparities.

So to summarize, decades before our current push to reduce costs and improve care under a population health model, cancer care was on the frontier of achieving just those goals. Not only did survival rates improve, but better early detection also meant a need for less chemotherapy and surgery to save money. Thanks to nurse navigators, many cancer patients have just one phone call to make.

The Principles of Patient Navigation[18]

There is much we can learn and apply to engagement by studying some of the foundational principles of patient navigation. For one thing, it is a patient-centric healthcare service delivery model built upon a trust-based relationship. That's just so important to the caregiver relationship as we have seen in the engagement model described earlier.

The focus is on outreach into the communities where patients live and to promote connections to the clinician for better access, greater timeliness, and improved outcomes from diagnosis to treatment and rehabilitation. It also serves as a way to virtually integrate care that would otherwise feel fragmented to patients.

It's important to understand that at its core, the function of the navigator is to eliminate barriers to receiving timely care across the healthcare continuum. The role of the navigator is distinct from that of other clinicians and yet integrated into the healthcare team. As a result, they serve as an important way to augment the impact of the clinical care team.

It's also designed to be a cost-effective role that aligns with the training and skills required to navigate a patient through a particular phase of care. So in some instances, a layperson will be effective as part of the team. In fact, the wife of a friend of mine was recently diagnosed with breast cancer and he shared their deep gratitude for this very role.

He told me that they had traveled out of state to a well-known cancer center, arriving anxious and frightened by his wife's diagnosis and wondering about the outcome and potential side effects of treatments. But what impressed them even more than the doctors or technology they experienced there were the volunteers in the reception areas who were all former patients. It was so comforting to have a "peer" sit beside them in the waiting area expressing empathy from a shared experience. This can be invaluable to patients.

Ideally, care navigators have backgrounds in a discipline such as nursing or social work. The goal is to match the education, experience, and skill level of the navigator who is selected to the sophistication of decisions and patient care that need to be provided. Also, within a given system of care, it's important to define the point when navigation begins and ends and for the navigator to oversee all phases of activity within a given site or system, particularly across disconnected systems like primary and tertiary care sites.

One best practice we can learn from what is used in breast cancer care is to create "protected" times in the schedule by blocking daily slots for additional diagnostic testing so patients can return as quickly as they desire, even the same day. Nurse navigators—who have insight into a woman's needs and emotions—can even schedule patients directly if the scheduling system is modified to allow it. By also offering immediate follow-up and prompt, personalized education and coaching, organizations can close perceived gaps in a patient's care.[19]

One best practice we can learn from what is used in breast cancer care is to create "protected" times in the schedule by blocking daily slots for additional diagnostic testing so patients can return as quickly as they desire.

In one study of the return on investment of nurse navigators in cancer care, researchers noted many positive outcomes after implementing a comprehensive navigation program.[20] The health system they studied dramatically improved patient retention, from 240 patients leaving annually pre-navigator implementation to just four patients four years after implementation. Other benefits included reduced patient anxiety and treatment delays; more timely access to healthcare and related resources; greater patient satisfaction; and empowered, shared decision-making education, which positively impacted patient choices and decisions.

Contrast these results with the experience of cancer care patients without access to nurse navigators. A woman without access to a navigator is more likely to experience fragmented care where she does a lot of waiting for results and appointments. The surgeon and oncologist may not be on the same page. Meanwhile, a woman with a nurse navigator can often be seen for a suspicious lump within 24 hours and be called with quick results, next steps, and scheduled for follow-up appointments.

Reinventing Healthcare

While nurse navigators represent a substantial improvement over anything else being used widely in the industry today to truly put patients at the center of their care, this approach doesn't go far enough. Think back to the earlier discussion about the simplicity of the user interface for an iPhone.

The enormous technological savvy required to conjure up a song on your phone in a split-second is incredibly sophisticated, but all of that complexity is in the background to the user, who doesn't even need an instruction manual these days to figure out how to navigate their phone. My vision is to see this level of true customer-centric design in our healthcare system.

In the meantime, we're fortunate to have skilled and caring navigators help us create a "virtual" system so that we can focus less on learning how to navigate our care systems, and more on the only thing that matters: our health.

But that isn't to say there aren't some places already headed toward this new reality. We can take inspiration about what the future of patient engagement looks like from several organizations that are successfully designing creative patient-centric solutions today.

Stanford Medicine in Northern California is one of them. It's working on reinventing the model for caring for patients with chronic illnesses.[21] Beginning in 2012, Dr. Alan Glaseroff, a family physician recognized nationally for his work in improving healthcare delivery and clinical professor of medicine at Stanford, opened an innovative new clinic based on a patient-centered intensive primary care model. The clinic offers team-based focused care with 24-hour availability, home visits, and regular support and coaching in self-management to Stanford Hospital employees and their families.

As someone who was diagnosed with type 1 diabetes himself years ago, he is particularly sensitive to his patients' fears around becoming disabled and their desire to take care of themselves and control their futures. "It's 2:00 in the morning, and you have a symptom. Either you panic and go to the emergency room or you have the skills to figure out what to do on your own," he explains. "You have someone you can call for advice, and you may resolve it or decide to go to the doctor's office in the morning. It's all about empowering people to make their own decisions."[22]

Glaseroff, who piloted a similar approach with Boeing's employees in Seattle, has developed an approach where his staff acts like an intensive care team but focuses on primary care (essentially acting as extensivists). The team includes health coaches who will visit patients at home, nurse practitioners who are available around the clock, a pharmacist, health educator, psychologist, and more. Dedicated medical specialists are also available to consult with patients.

A similar approach is also being used at Kaiser San Rafael Medical Center, also in the Bay Area, in its PHASE—or Preventing Heart Attack and Stroke Every Day—program.[23] Because cardiovascular disease is the leading cause of death and disability in the United States, the program's goal is to identify patients early, educate them, and monitor them closely. They are very intentional about their goal of ensuring that patients perceive their doctor and nurses as a trusted team.

PHASE patients are referred by primary care physicians as part of secondary prevention for myocardial infarction, coronary heart disease, diabetes, peripheral vascular disease, or stroke. Then they are co-managed by specially trained pharmacist care managers who work directly with the patient and his doctor in the doctor's office.

As Dr. Dan Smith, a family physician at Kaiser San Rafael says, "The program works. It has lowered the likelihood of death due to heart disease by 30 percent. If you are a Northern California Kaiser member, your risk of dying from heart disease is lower than your risk of dying from cancer."[24]

Are these programs perfect? Surely not. The weak link in the PHASE program is its dependence upon connecting with primary care doctors who will enroll patients. Funding is also a challenge with upfront costs for uncertain pay-offs later.

And yet, the healthcare industry must find a way to move away from funding sick care to investing in wellness programs like these if it's to succeed in the years ahead. Examples like these are moving us in the right direction.

Whether it's navigators, coaches, or even technology, anything that puts patients first is a welcome improvement. In the years to come, I look forward to learning more from organizations that are truly redesigning systems and processes that put complexity and inefficiency firmly in the background of the patient experience.

Key Learning Points: Beyond the Caregiver—The Role of Technology and Organizational Design in Patient Engagement

1. Collecting and recording psychosocial data, PAM scores, information about health literacy, and a patient's personal health goals are powerful ways to identify common barriers to engagement that can be addressed one patient at a time.

2. While technology will never be an effective substitute for an informed and compassionate caregiver, it can add much value when used as a tool to support higher patient engagement.

3. Telehealth is growing quickly and is embraced by a majority of patients.

4. Designing a patient-centric organization starts with the voice of the customer. While the nurse navigator model demonstrates the potential return on investment for organizations that make patient engagement easier, the healthcare industry is still in its infancy of designing truly patient-centric organizations. The goal is to make the system so easy to use that navigators are unnecessary.

CONCLUSION

Hopefully, this book has made a compelling case for the critical role that engagement will play in transforming healthcare and given you a sense of some tools you can use to increase engagement in your organization. And now the hard part...actually doing it!

As you get ready to do just that, I'd like to leave you with two final thoughts: First, how to be an engaged patient yourself. And second, how to help others engage.

Be an Engaged Patient Yourself[1]

Unfortunately, each of us will likely have opportunities in the years to come to appreciate the patient perspective as we access healthcare for ourselves or people we love. In that spirit, I'd like to share several tips consistent with current evidence that each of us can use to take ownership of our own engagement as a patient or family member.

One of the most important things you can do is to share feedback with the organizations you visit so they can be better for the next patient. Commit to completing and returning any survey you receive after your visit.

Consider going the extra mile with a written letter to the clinic or hospital you visited to share what went well, who was helpful, and what could be improved. If you experienced a serious problem with quality or safety, follow up to see if it was resolved. Because if we don't speak up, we become complicit in perpetuating the problem.

Never underestimate the power of these letters. I recently spoke to a group of healthcare leaders where one of the participants was an executive at a hospital where Julie's dad received great care. When I mentioned her name, he immediately remembered us. "Oh, she's the one who wrote that great letter," he said immediately. "We've read that note to all of the staff. It was so appreciated."

Also, be an active information-seeker. Engaged patients are prepared patients. So seek out information online or at the library to understand your symptoms or treatment choices. But also remember that Google is no replacement for the skill of a trained diagnostician who can cull through the infinite information available to identify the facts relevant to your situation.

Invite your care provider into this partnering process by asking about recommended websites or apps. Then prepare for your next visit by writing down any important information and questions ahead of time.

In the same vein, keep a record of your medical files and review it. If your physician uses an electronic patient portal, take advantage of it. Always ask for a copy of the visit summary and any tests that were completed before you leave. Ask for clarity about how lab test results will be shared. Speak up if you usually get blue pills, but this time they were red. Remember, you serve as an important safety check through your consistent and proactive efforts to validate the quality of your care.

Consider volunteering as a patient and family advisor at your local clinic or hospital. There's just no substitute for a patient's perspective and experience as organizations strive to reinvent themselves to put patients first. If you learn that the organization doesn't work with patient and family advisors, ask them to consider doing so.

Finally, be sure to take your medications as directed. (Don't save the remaining antibiotics even though you're feeling better!) Keep your appointments and do the things we all know we should to stay healthy: stop smoking or don't start, watch your weight and what you eat, stay current with immunizations and routine tests, wash your hands regularly, and exercise.

But it's not enough to just be engaged patients ourselves. To truly transform our industry, we need to activate everyone we work with. Radiate your engagement to others around you.

Help Others Engage

Over the past decade, I've been privileged to work with literally hundreds of organizations and tens of thousands of healthcare leaders. And I've found that what sets apart the best from the rest is the ability to connect with people in a way that touches upon our shared values. If you want to engage people in your work or personal life, master this skill.

If you're familiar with Studer Group®, you know that we coach leaders on the importance of explaining the *why* behind the *what* of what we ask people to do. It helps us to connect back to our desire for a sense of purpose in our work. But I've found that there's a bit more to it than that. I believe we really need to touch upon *three* levels of *why*—the head, the heart, and what's in it for me—to ensure our message is heard deeply and anchored in a person's values.

> **We really need to touch upon *three* levels of *why*—the head, the heart, and what's in it for me.**

The first level of *why*—the head—satisfies our rational need for logical thought and evidence that's conveyed by data, best practices, and large sample sizes. But as my colleague Dr. Gurpreet Dhaliwal says, "Nobody has ever taken to the streets because of a pie chart!"

To motivate people, we need to connect with them on an emotional level. That's the heart, the second level of *why*. In fact, there's mounting evidence that most of the decisions we make are not based on logic, but, rather, on emotion. An emotion isn't ever conveyed with data. It's conveyed through compelling stories…not an N of 300 or more, but, rather, an N of just one.

What's still missing from this concept, though, is the third level of *why*—making it personal: What's in it for me? How does this make my life better, easier, more productive, or efficient? I'm busy; why should I do this particular thing right now rather than the 70 other pressing items? How does it address the core reasons why I went into this profession 20 years ago? Think of this one as the N of *me*.

If you can craft a message that touches the head, the heart, and what's in it for me, I guarantee that you will be much more likely to compel people to engage in whatever it is you're hoping to promote. I've found it's helpful to explain this concept through an example. Since most audiences I work with are very familiar with AIDET®, this works nicely.

Back when I joined Studer Group a decade ago as the leader of research and development, I was convinced that if I shared 30 or 40 slides with impressive quantitative data about the impact of AIDET—and there is great data—that I could declare victory. I just had to put the evidence into smart people's heads and they would go do it, right?

Explaining the *why of the head* was the only one I'd been formally trained to discuss and the only one I thought I needed to master. (Of course, that's not the case. If data and evidence were all we needed, no one would smoke and we would each exercise 30 minutes a day!)

But then I was given a gift that helped me to understand the reason that we really use AIDET. And ultimately, this is what it looked like:

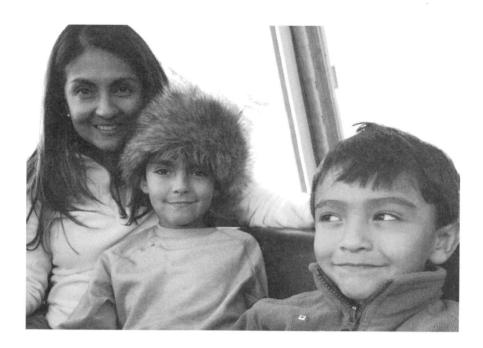

That's my wife, Julie, and my two sons, Sam and Jack. Let's rewind the clock ten years. Soon after Julie and I relocated from Dallas to Pensacola, Florida, for my new job at Studer Group, we learned that Julie was pregnant. (When I share this story in my talks, I used to say that we learned that *"we"* were pregnant, but my predominately female audiences pointed out that I was never pregnant. Good point!)

We were both very anxious about this pregnancy because we'd experienced two prior miscarriages. (And those were definitely a "we.") Julie actually flew back to Dallas to consult with her OB because she was so anxious. They'd developed such a bond through the two prior pregnancies and had shared a lot.

Julie was treated as a whole person by that physician. But ultimately, he wisely pointed out the limitations of prenatal care by airplane, so Julie soon found a great OB in Pensacola, who referred her to a specialist since her pregnancy was so high-risk. Soon thereafter, Julie and I sat anxiously waiting in an exam room to meet this new specialist.

After about ten minutes, a young woman entered. She was wearing scrubs with a white coat. There was some stitching on her jacket, which we presumed to be her name, but we couldn't read it because her hair covered it and her name badge was twisted around backward. (So I was able to read about what happens if there's a Code Blue, which is nice to know as a safety-focused person, but I didn't catch any details about her role.)

She began by saying, "Hi. My name is Stephanie *(fictionalized)*." Then she opened up Julie's medical record and began asking very personal questions about her medical history. I don't know if you've been present for someone else's history, but it was pretty uncomfortable.

I noticed that Julie seemed uncomfortable, too, as her responses became less detailed and more guarded. On one occasion, I felt she was leaving out some pretty important facts and I figured my presence was inhibiting her candor, so I offered to step out. But Julie said, "No, I'd really prefer it if you stayed."

Julie continued to answer questions, monosyllabically, for another few minutes until Stephanie said, "Craig, I understand you moved here for your job. What do you do?" So I told her that I worked for a small local company called Studer Group.

Stephanie's eyes widened and she broke out into a big smile of recognition. I started to relax for a moment, thinking things were about to improve. But that feeling lasted all of ten seconds. Because next, she stood up, closed Julie's medical record, and left the room without a single word. You can imagine our utter confusion!

About 20 seconds later we heard a knock at the door, and Stephanie walked back in. Her lab coat was buttoned professionally. Her hair was pulled back and her name badge had been adjusted. Then she said, "Hi. My name is Stephanie Alexander. I'm a double master's-prepared genetics counselor and I've been working with Dr. Smith *(fictionalized)* in his practice for the last seven years.

"Between the two of us, we've been privileged to provide help and hope to hundreds of people who come to us from all over the Gulf Coast region. I'm delighted to be able to spend this time with you today.

"I know you said you hadn't met Dr. Smith yet, but not only are his outcomes phenomenal, but he's just a great guy. You'll get to see that for yourself because in about 20 minutes you will meet him down the hall in a conference room where you can ask him any questions you've got on your minds and talk about the course of care from there."

She continued: "Let me explain what I'm going to be doing over these next 20 minutes. I'm going to be asking you a series of history questions. While 20 minutes may seem longer than you've experienced for past histories, it's important because all of this information will be used to form a risk profile that will ultimately recommend how frequently you'll be seen in the practice and determine the types of tests and intensity of treatments to produce the best possible outcome for your family.

"I apologize if I don't always make good eye contact while I enter your responses into the medical record. I'm listening, but I don't want to miss any of this important information for Dr. Smith."

Then Stephanie smirked slightly and said in a saccharine tone, "Oh, but I'm not done. Let me not miss the opportunity to say *thank you*." Then she unbuttoned her coat, dropped the file folder back on the chair and laughed.

What just happened?! We were confused. She'd just delivered an excellent AIDET, but why did she laugh at the end? Why did she seem so sarcastic?

"I just thought you'd get a kick out of that because you said you worked at Studer Group," she explained. "A few weeks ago, our boss played your AIDET video so we all had to write our little AIDET scripts. See? Here's mine right here!" (Pause the story: If someone calls this a "script," have they really internalized why it's a meaningful communication practice?)

"It was great," I told her. Then I asked: "But why don't you do that for every patient and not just those who work at Studer Group?"

"To be honest, it's kind of uncomfortable for me," she answered.

And then Julie responded. She said, "Stephanie, this clears up a few things. First of all, I thought you were Dr. Stephanie Smith. And, I have to be honest, I'd already fired you in my mind a few minutes after you began asking me questions. This is the hardest thing I've been through in my life now...for the third time.

"What made the last two miscarriages a little easier was the incredible relationship I had with my doctor in Dallas. I wasn't feeling that with you. I was already thinking about how to get out of here and where to look next for another specialist. But from what you said, this doctor sounds great."

She added, "Now that I understand that all of this information I'm sharing is going to guide that risk profile, there are some other things I want to make sure you include in the chart for Dr. Smith." And then Julie proceeded to give more detail in areas where I thought she'd been too quick to cover previously.

I noticed that Stephanie wrote those things down. So I asked her if she felt they were clinically relevant and helpful. "Yes," she responded.

I asked her if they could change Julie's risk profile. "Well, it could," she answered. So I confirmed with her that that additional information would determine tests and treatments and possibly even the *outcome* for our family. She agreed.

"So, to paraphrase," I paraphrased, "if I hear you right, Stephanie, you're saying AIDET isn't something you do to raise a patient's satisfaction score or just to comply with what the boss says. Rather, it's part of a good clinical encounter that builds a trusting relationship with a patient so that you can capture a full and complete history. So actually, AIDET is part of creating good outcomes for patients."

And Stephanie said, "I guess I never thought of it like that before." When I asked her if she'd use it from now on for all of her patients, she said she wasn't sure…because it wasn't comfortable for her.

I was angry at the time. I was less concerned about her comfort than the comfort of her patient, my wife. If there is something she could say to make Julie more comfortable and get a better outcome, then that has to become an *always* behavior for every patient, every time.

At times we *must* do things that are uncomfortable if they're best for the patient. Caregivers do it every day when they share difficult news or support their patients through a challenging procedure.

Nine months after the visit to that specialist, Julie and I felt like we won the lottery when she gave birth to Sam, who is now nine. And a few years after that, our son Jack.

So that's the *why of the heart* for AIDET. I've been privileged to share this story hundreds of times and I've been surprised at the impact it's made. At one event, a CEO even approached me and said, "I saw you give this talk back in January and wondered if you were planning to tell the story about your wife again today."

I sheepishly responded that I was, and that I'd understand if he wanted to attend another session since he'd already heard it. But then he said, "No, the reason I'm asking is that I've brought six members of my team today hoping you'd share this story, because I think it will help them understand why we're doing all of these practices in the first place."

I was blown away. And so, since that day, every time I'm given the opportunity, I've shared this story about the *why of the heart* in case others benefit in the same way.

Now, can you guess how many people came up to me before I spoke and asked if I was going to show a certain data slide again because they felt it would have such an impact on their teammates? Zero.

The *why of the heart* is always more compelling than the *why of the head*. But to really bring it home, don't forget to touch the final base: *what's in it for me*. For AIDET, that's easy. When I take the time to acknowledge someone in my presence, explain who I am, what I'm about to do and why, I see the impact it has on them. Put simply: When I'm nice to people, they're nice back to me.

So I encourage you: As you lean into engagement in the months and years to come, take a moment to build out a message that touches on all three levels of *why*: the head, the heart, and the what's in it for me.

In that same spirit, I hope the evidence and the stories in this book helped *you* re-engage and will light a fire to help others on the same journey in the years to come. I look forward to hearing your stories.

ACKNOWLEDGMENTS

How did I get so lucky? For the past decade, I've been privileged to work with the most passionate and interesting people in healthcare, inside one of the most widely celebrated companies in the industry, doing work that I love.

Thank you, first, to my colleagues at Studer Group and Huron. Not only does our coaching transform lives and organizations, we also have this remarkable national platform where we can develop and share ideas around the world through our speaking, conferences, and publishing teams. BG and Debbie, your leadership and friendship over the past ten years have been major influences on my own level of engagement. And I have special appreciation for our coaches, fellow speakers, and hundreds of teammates who share the same passion I do to make healthcare better for employees, physicians, and patients.

Several times over the months writing this book I thought of Jack Nicholson's character in *The Shining*. On the one hand, I empathize with his idea of holing up in a mountain retreat for a few months to finally write his book. At times, that seemed like a much more efficient process. But then I remembered how that ended up for him in the movie and quickly realized how grateful I am for the enormous talent who did the heavy lifting for this book, especially Chris Roman, whose personal engagement in this book was the only way it was finally written; Lindy Sikes, for helping us stay on track; Lauren Westwood, who helps people see the things I only envision in my mind; and the team at DeHart & Company for bringing yet another book to life with our team.

Before I felt confident to put pen to paper, I became a student of engagement. My teachers were the audiences in hundreds of organizations where I've spoken, the papers I read, and the dozens of personal discussions with true experts on various topics in the book, most especially Dr. Judith Hibbard, Dave Fox, Patrick Bucknum, Dr. Gurpreet Dhaliwal, Debbie Ritchie, Don Dean, Jeff Jones, Gary Anthony, Faye Sullivan, Dr. Rob Schreiner, Vikki Choate, Dr. Jeff Morris, Dr. Dan Smith, Julie O'Shaughnessy, Hazel Seabrook, Dr. Ted James, Karen Fraser, Marty Hatlie, Andy Ziskind, Dr. Larry Magras, and Ted Schwab.

Everyone thinks of changing the world, but no one thinks of changing himself. I close just about every presentation with this quote from Tolstoy. Not only does it nicely sum up most of the messages I deliver, but it also reminds me, as I travel home, to practice with my family what I just taught to others. Speaking of engagement, Julie, thank you for saying "yes" twelve years ago! Your edits made this book better; our relationship makes my life better. Sam and Jack, I can't wait to see how you'll change the world. Mom and Dad, thank you for showing me what great parents do; our boys are lucky to have you in their lives.

Finally, I want to thank my mother-in-law, Mari, who allowed me to share Jaime's personal story. Her courage and strength in the face of a devastating life event have been an inspiration and comfort to her children and her grandchildren. To my parents and our close friends, Phil and Pam Hall and Robyn and Scott Christensen, who took in our children and offered them a comforting home when I was traveling and Julie was with her dad, thank you. Without their acts of kindness and their support, Julie would not have been able to be away from our young family for that amount of time. It afforded her precious time with her father, moments for which we will always be grateful.

REFERENCES

Part 1:

1. Pfeffer, Jeffrey, and Robert I. Sutton. *The Knowing-Doing Gap: How Smart Companies Turn Knowledge into Action*. Boston: Harvard Business School Press, 2000.

2. Gruman, Jessie, Margaret Holmes Rovner, Molly E. French, Dorothy Jeffress, Shoshanna Sofaer, Dale Shaller, and Denis J. Prager. "From Patient Education to Patient Engagement: Implications for the Field of Patient Education." *Patient Education & Counseling* 78 no. 3 (2010): 350-356. Accessed July 13, 2016. doi: http://dx.doi.org/10.1016/j.pec.2010.02.002.

3. Gallup, Inc. "State of the Global Workplace." Accessed August 1, 2016. http://www.gallup.com/services/178517/state-global-workplace.aspx.

4. Parekh, Anand K. "Winning Their Trust." *New England Journal of Medicine* 364, no. 24 (2011): e51. doi: 10.1056/NEJMp1105645.

5. Akerlof, George A. "Procrastination and Obedience." *The American Economic Review* 81, no. 2 (1991): 1-19. http://www.jstor.org/stable/2006817.

6. Parekh, Anand K. "Winning Their Trust." *New England Journal of Medicine* 364, no. 24 (2011): e51. doi: 10.1056/NEJMp1105645.

7. Ibid

8. Shrank William H., Niteesh K. Choudhry, Michael A. Fischer, Jerry Avorn, Mark Powell, Sebastian Schneeweis, Joshua N. Liberman, Timothy Dollear, Troyen A. Brennan, and M. Alan Brookhart. "The Epidemiology of Prescriptions Abandoned at the Pharmacy." *Annals of Internal*

Medicine 153, no. 10 (2010): 633-640. doi:10.7326/0003-4819-153-10-201011160-00005

9. U.S. Department of Health and Human Services. "Prevention Makes Common Cents." Accessed June 14, 2016. https://aspe.hhs.gov/legacy-page/prevention-makes-common-cent-142526.

Chapter 1:

1. Linzer, Mark, Rachel Levine, David Meltzer, Sara Poplau, Carole Warde, and Colin P. West. "10 Bold Steps to Prevent Burnout in General Internal Medicine." *Journal of General Internal Medicine* 29, no. 1 (2014): 18-20. doi:10.1007/s11606-013-2597-8.

2. Tobacco Use and Dependence Guideline Panel. *Treating Tobacco Use and Dependence: 2008 Update.* Rockville: US Department of Health and Human Services, 2008. http://www.ncbi.nlm.nih.gov/books/NBK63952/.

3. Burger, Jeff and Andrew Giger. "Want to Increase Hospital Revenues? Engage Your Physicians." *Gallup Business Journal* (2014). Accessed July 6, 2016. http://www.gallup.com/businessjournal/170786/increase-hospital-revenues-engage-physicians.aspx.

4. Hemp, Paul. "Presenteeism: At Work – But Out of It." *Harvard Business Review*, October 2004. Accessed June 17, 2016. https://hbr.org/2004/10/presenteeism-at-work-but-out-of-it.

5. Stewart, Walter F., Judith A. Ricci, Elsbeth Chee, Steven R. Hahn, and David Morganstein. "Cost of Lost Productive Work Time Among US Workers with Depression." *Journal of the American Medical Association* 289 no. 23 (2003): 3135-3144. doi: 10.1001/jama.289.23.3135.

6. Stewart Walter F., Judith A. Ricci, Elsbeth Chee, David Morganstein, and Richard Lipton. "Lost Productive Time and Cost Due to Common Pain Conditions in the US Workforce." *Journal of the American Medical Association* 290 no. 18 (2003): 2443-2454. doi: 10.1001/jama.290.18.2443.

7. Studer Group. "Preventable Readmissions: Focus on Improving Continuum of Care (Part 1 of 2)." March 25, 2013.

8. The Henry J. Kaiser Family Foundation. "2015 Employer Health Benefits Survey." September 22, 2015. http://kff.org/report-section/ehbs-2015-section-seven-employee-cost-sharing/.

9. Fronstin, Paul. "Findings from the 2013 EBRI/Greenwald & Associates Consumer Engagement in Health Care Survey." *EBRI Issue Brief*

no. 393 (2013). https://www.ebri.org/pdf/briefspdf/EBRI_IB_012-13. No393.CEHCS.pdf.

10. Dugan, Andrew. "Cost Still Delays Healthcare for About One in Three in U.S." Gallup, November 30, 2015. http://www.gallup.com/poll/187190/cost-delays-healthcare-one-three.aspx.

11. Rand Corporation. "Analysis of High Deductible Health Plans." Accessed June 17, 2016. http://www.rand.org/pubs/technical_reports/TR562z4/analysis-of-high-deductible-health-plans.html.

12. Sondra Cari, e-mail message to author, June 13, 2016.

13. Luhby, Tami. "Typical American family earned $53,657 last year." CNNMoney, September 16, 2015. http://money.cnn.com/2015/09/16/news/economy/census-poverty-income/.

14. Lamontagne, Christina. "NerdWallet Health Finds Medical Bankruptcy Accounts for Majority of Personal Bankruptcies." Nerdwallet, March 26, 2014. https://www.nerdwallet.com/blog/health/medical-bankruptcy/.

Chapter 2:

1. Schroeder, Steven A. "We Can Do Better – Improving the Health of the American People." *New England Journal of Medicine* 357 no. 12 (2007): 1221-1228. doi: 10.1056/NEJMsa073350.

2. Ofri, Danielle. "When the Patient is 'Noncompliant'." *Well* (blog), *New York Times*, November 15, 2012. http://well.blogs.nytimes.com/2012/11/15/when-the-patient-is-noncompliant/.

3. Steiner, John F. "Rethinking Adherence." *Annals of Internal Medicine* 157 no. 8 (2012): 580-585. doi: 10.7326/0003-4819-157-8-201210160-00013.

4. Ofri, Danielle. "When the Patient is 'Noncompliant'." *Well* (blog), *New York Times*, November 15, 2012. http://well.blogs.nytimes.com/2012/11/15/when-the-patient-is-noncompliant/.

5. Gary Anthony (managing director, Huron Healthcare), in discussion with the author, May 31, 2016.

6. Kotter, John P. and Dan S. Cohen. *The Heart of Change*. Boston, MA: Harvard Business Review Press, 2012.

7. Dave Fox (Chief Executive Officer, Advocate Good Samaritan Hospital), discussion with the author, July 1, 2016.

8. Worden, Ian. "Patient Experience vs. Patient Engagement." *Better Patient Engagement* (blog), July 15, 2012. http://www.betterpatientengagement.com/2012/07/15/patient-experience-vs-patient-engagement/ (site discontinued).

9. Worden, Ian. "Why Patient Experiences Should Foster Engagement." *Better Patient Engagement* (blog), September 2, 2014. http://www.betterpatientengagement.com/2014/09/02/patient-experiences-foster-engagement/ (site discontinued).

10. PRWeb. "Insignia Health Earns 'Best in Class' Endorsement from National Quality Forum for a Person and Family-Centered Care Measure." Press Release, June 6, 2016. http://www.prweb.com/releases/2016/06/prweb13466816.htm.

11. Gulsvig, Janice. "Patient activation and engagement," *McKnight's*, December 15, 2015, http://www.mcknights.com/marketplace/patient-activation-and-engagement/article/459663/.

12. Hibbard, Judith H., Jessica Greene, and Valerie Overton. "Patients with Lower Activation Associated with Higher Costs; Delivery Systems Should Know Their Patients' 'Scores'." *Health Affairs* 32 no. 2 (2013): 216-222 doi: 10.1377/hlthaff.2012.1064.

13. Ibid

14. Ibid

15. Ibid

16. Winner, Brooke, Jeffrey F. Peipert, Qiuhong Zhao, Christina Buckel, Tessa Madden, Jennifer E. Allsworth, and Gina M. Secura. "Effectiveness of Long-Acting Reversible Contraception." *New England Journal of Medicine* 366 no. 21 (2012): 1998–2007. doi: 10.1056/NEJMoa1110855.

17. Judith Hibbard, interview with the author, July 7, 2016.

18. Rigoni, J. Brandon and Bailey Nelson. "The No-Managers Organizational Approach Doesn't Work." *Gallup Business Journal*, February 5, 2016, http://www.gallup.com/businessjournal/189074/no-managers-organizational-approach-doesn-work.aspx?utm_source=genericbutton&utm_medium=organic&utm_campaign=sharing.

19. Wagner, Rodd and Jim Harter. "The First Element of Great Managing." *Gallup Business Journal*, February 8, 2007, http://www.gallup.com/businessjournal/26281/First-Element-Great-Managing.aspx.

20. Ibid

21. Chase, David. "Is There a Business Case for Patient Engagement?" *The Health Care Blog*, March 4, 2015. http://thehealthcareblog.com/blog/2015/03/04/is-there-a-business-case-for-patient-engagement/.

Chapter 3:

1. Daugherty, Alicia. "What Do Consumers Want from Primary Care?" Advisory Board, June 25, 2014. https://www.advisory.com/Research/Market-Innovation-Center/expert-insights/2014/get-the-primary-care-consumer-choice-survey-results.
2. Ibid
3. Young, Jeffrey. "Why We're Picking Walmart and CVS Over Doctors' Offices." *Huffington Post*, January 12, 2015, http://www.huffingtonpost.com/2015/01/12/retail-clinics_n_6445506.html.
4. Ibid
5. Frost & Sullivan. "Retail Healthcare Transforms Patients Seek Alternative Healthcare Options Driving Growth Opportunities for Traditional and Non-Traditional Care Givers." Press Release, June 7, 2016. http://ww2.frost.com/news/press-releases/retail-healthcare-transforms-patients-seek-alternative-healthcare-options-driving-growth-opportunities-traditional-and-non-tradi/.
6. Young, Jeffrey. "Why We're Picking Walmart and CVS Over Doctors' Offices." The Huffington Post, January 12, 2015. http://www.huffingtonpost.com/2015/01/12/retail-clinics_n_6445506.html.
7. Association of American Medical Colleges. "New Research Confirms Looming Physician Shortage." Press Release, April, 5, 2016. https://www.aamc.org/newsroom/newsreleases/458074/2016_workforce_projections_04052016.html.
8. Ibid
9. Duhigg, Charles. "How Companies Learn Your Secrets." *New York Times Magazine*, February 16, 2012. http://www.nytimes.com/2012/02/19/magazine/shopping-habits.html?pagewanted=1&_r=2&hp.
10. Appleby, Julie. "Walgreens Becomes 1st Retail Chain to Diagnose, Treat Chronic Conditions." *Kaiser Health News*, April 4, 2013, http://khn.org/news/walgreens-primary-care-services/.
11. Berthiaume, Dan. "CVS Health's New Digital Innovation Lab Focuses on Customer Experience." *Chain Store Age*, June 18, 2015, http://www.

chainstoreage.com/article/cvs-health%E2%80%99s-new-digital-innovation-lab-focuses-customer-experience.

12. Ibid

13. Target Corporation. "Target Clinic: Your One-Stop-Shop for Health and Wellness." November 17, 2014. https://corporate.target.com/article/2014/11/target-clinic.

14. Sun, Lena H. "Haven't Got Your Flu Shot? Uber is Offering One-Day, On-Demand Vaccinations to Your Doorstep." *Washington Post*, November 17, 2015. https://www.washingtonpost.com/news/to-your-health/wp/2015/11/17/no-time-to-get-your-flu-shot-uber-is-offering-on-demand-vaccinations-to-your-doorstep/.

15. Ibid

16. Gawande, Atul. *Being Mortal.* New York: Metropolitan Books, 2014.

17. Bodel, Lisa. *Kill the Company: End the Status Quo, Start an Innovation Revolution.* Brookline: Bibliomotion, 2012. Page 50.

Part 3:

1. Studer, Quint. *Hardwired Results* 13 (2013): 2-3. https://www.studergroup.com/hardwiredresults13.

Chapter 4:

1. HR Solutions, Inc. "Study Reveals Near-Perfect Pearson Correlation Between Hand Washing and Employee Engagement". Press Release, November 30, 2010. https://www.prlog.org/11113465-study-reveals-near-perfect-pearson-correlation-between-hand-washing-and-employee-engagement.html.

2. Nystrom, Bertil. "Impact of Handwashing on Mortality in Intensive Care: Examination of the Evidence." *Infection Control & Hospital Epidemiology* 15 no. 7 (1994): 435-436.

3. Reybrouck, G. "Role of hands in the spread of nosocomial infections." *Journal of Hospital Infection* 4 no. 2 (1983): 103-110. doi: http://dx.doi.org/10.1016/0195-6701(83)90040-3.

4. Pittet, Didier. "Improving Adherence to Hand Hygiene Practice: A Multidisciplinary Approach." *Emerging Infectious Diseases Journal* 7 no.2 (2001). doi: 10.3201/eid0702.700234.

5. HR Solutions, Inc. "Study Reveals Near-Perfect Pearson Correlation Between Hand Washing and Employee Engagement". Press Release, November 30, 2010. https://www.prlog.org/11113465-study-reveals-near-perfect-pearson-correlation-between-hand-washing-and-employee-engagement.html.

6. Studer, Quint. "Selecting and Retaining Talent: Tools for the Bottom Line." *Healthcare Financial Management*, July 2006.

7. Hotko, Barbara. "Rounding for Outcomes: How to Increase Employee Retention and Drive Higher Patient Satisfaction." *Hardwired Results* 1 (2004): 4-8. https://www.studergroup.com/hardwiredresults01.

8. Rigoni, J. Brandon and Bailey Nelson. "The No-Managers Organizational Approach Doesn't Work." Gallup Business Journal, February 5, 2016, http://www.gallup.com/businessjournal/189074/no-managers-organizational-approach-doesn-work.aspx?utm_source=genericbutton&utm_medium=organic&utm_campaign=sharing.

9. Ibid

10. Ibid

11. Ibid

12. Studer, Quint. *Hardwiring Excellence*, 38. Pensacola: Fire Starter Publishing, 2003.

13. Buckingham, Marcus and Curt Coffman. *First Break All the Rules: What the World's Greatest Managers Do Differently*. New York: Simon & Schuster, 1999.

Chapter 5:

1. Cejka Search and AMGA. "2013 Physician Retention Survey." April 19, 2013

2. Smith, Dan. "The Hidden Costs of Declining Physician Engagement." Hardwired Results 14 (2014): 5. https://www.studergroup.com/hardwiredresults14.

3. Linzer, Mark, Linda Baier Manwell, Marlon Mundt, Eric Williams, Ann Maguire, Julia McMurray, and Mary Beth Plane. "Organizational Climate, Stress, and Error in Primary Care: The MEMO Study." In Advances in Patient Safety: From Research to Implementation. Vol. 1, Research Findings, edited by Kerm Henriksen, James B. Battles, Eric S.

Marks, and David I. Lewin. Rockville: Agency for Healthcare Research and Quality, 2005.

4. Ibid

5. Quantia. "Physicians Reveal the Kind of Leader They Will – and Won't – Follow." Accessed November 6, 2014. http://www.quantia-inc.com/physicians-reveal-kind-leader-will-wont-follow/ (page discontinued).

6. Ibid

7. Amabile, Teresa and Steven J. Kramer. "The Power of Small Wins." Harvard Business Review, May 2011. https://hbr.org/2011/05/the-power-of-small-wins.

8. Studer, Quint. Healing Physician Burnout, 146. Pensacola: Fire Starter Publishing, 2015.

9. Ibid

10. Studer, Quint. Healing Physician Burnout, 104-107 and 119-120. Pensacola: Fire Starter Publishing, 2015.

11. Studer Group. "Physician Collaboration Toolkit." 2007.

12. Huron Consulting Group. "Physician Selection Toolkit."2016.

13. Greene, Jessica, Judith H. Hibbard, Carmen Alvarez, and Valerie Overton. "Supporting Patient Behavior Change: Approaches Used by Primary Care Clinicians Whose Patients Have an Increase in Activation Levels." Annals of Family Medicine 14 no. 2 (2016): 148-154.

14. Alvarez, Carmen, Jessica Greene, Judith Hibbard, and Valerie Overton. "The Role of Primary Care Providers in Patient Activation and Engagement in Self-Management: A Cross-Sectional Analysis." BMC Health Services Research 16 no. 1 (2016): 1-8. doi: 10.1186/s12913-016-1328-3.

15. Hibbard, Judith H., Peter Alf Collins, Eldon Mahoney, and Laurence H. Baker. "The Development and Testing of a Measure Assessing Clinician Beliefs About Patient Self-Management." Health Expectations 13 no. 1 (2010): 65-72. doi: 10.1111/j.1369-7625.2009.00571.x.

16. Alvarez, Carmen, Jessica Greene, Judith Hibbard, and Valerie Overton. "The Role of Primary Care Providers in Patient Activation and Engagement in Self-Management: A Cross-Sectional Analysis." BMC Health Services Research 16 no. 1 (2016): 1-8. doi: 10.1186/s12913-016-1328-3.

17. Studer Group. "Physician Collaboration Toolkit." 2007.

Chapter 6:

1. Makoul, Gregory, Amanda Zick, and Marianne Green. "An Evidence-Based Perspective on Greetings in Medical Encounters." Archives of Internal Medicine 167 no. 11 (2007): 1172 – 1176. doi: 10.1001/archinte.167.11.1172.

2. Greene, Jessica, Judith H. Hibbard, Carmen Alvarez, and Valerie Overton. "Supporting Patient Behavior Change: Approaches Used by Primary Care Clinicians Whose Patients Have an Increase in Activation Levels." Annals of Family Medicine 14 no. 2 (2016): 148-154.

3. Meade, Chris, Amy Bursell, and Lyn Ketelsen. "Effects of Nursing Rounds: On Patients' Call Light Use, Satisfaction, and Safety." American Journal of Nursing 106 no. 9 (2006): 58-71.

4. Collard, Dan. "Reduce Falls, Overtime and Lost Charges with Hourly Rounding." Hardwired Results 8 (2007): 7. https://www.studergroup.com/hardwired-results/hardwired-results-08/reduce-falls-overtime-and-lost-charges.

5. Ibid

6. Deao, Craig. "Patient-Centered Care: Engagement Matters." Hardwired Results 19 (2015): 5. https://www.studergroup.com/hardwiredresults19.

7. James, Julia. "Health Policy Brief: Patient Engagement." Health Affairs, February 14, 2013. http://www.healthaffairs.org/healthpolicybriefs/brief.php?brief_id=86.

8. Studer Group. "Reducing No-Shows Takes a Personal Touch." Insights (blog), February 23, 2015. https://www.studergroup.com/resources/news-media/healthcare-publications-resources/insights/february-2015/reducing-no-shows-takes-a-personal-touch.

9. Prachyl, Dianna. "7 Ways to Improve Access and Reduce No-Shows." Hardwired Results 14 (2014): 8-9. https://www.studergroup.com/hardwiredresults14.

10. Studer Group. "Increase Access with Pre-Visit Phone Calls." Hardwired Results 3 (2005): 7. https://www.studergroup.com/hardwiredresults03.

11. Ibid

12. Hazel Seabrook (managing director, Huron Healthcare), in discussion with the author, August, 19, 2016.

13. "It's a Dog's World, 2nd Edition." CRM Learning video, 14:00. http://www.crmlearning.com/It-s-a-Dog-s-World-C8783-P54513.aspx.

14. Forester, Alan J., Harvey J. Murff, Josh F. Peterson, Tejal K. Gandhi, and David W. Bates. "The Incidence and Severity of Adverse Events Affecting Patients after Discharge from the Hospital." Annals of Internal Medicine 138 no. 3 (2003): 161-167. doi: 10.7326/0003-4819-138-3-200302040-00007.

15. Hibbard, Judith H., Peter Alf Collins, Eldon Mahoney, and Laurence H. Baker. "The Development and Testing of a Measure Assessing Clinician Beliefs About Patient Self-Management." Health Expectations 13 no. 1 (2010): 65-72. doi: 10.1111/j.1369-7625.2009.00571.x.

16. James, Julia. "Health Policy Brief: Patient Engagement." Health Affairs, February 14, 2013. http://www.healthaffairs.org/healthpolicybriefs/brief.php?brief_id=86.

17. Swayden, Kelli J., Karen K. Anderson, Lynne M. Connelly, Jennifer S. Moran, Joan K. McMahon, and Paul M. Arnold. "Effect of Sitting vs. Standing on Perception of Provider Time at Bedside: A Pilot Study." Patient Education and Counseling 86 no. 2 (2012): 166-171. doi: http://dx.doi.org/10.1016/j.pec.2011.05.024.

18. Davis, Rachel E., M. Koutantji, and C.A. Vincent. "How Willing Are Patients to Question Healthcare Staff on Issues Related to the Quality and Safety of Their Healthcare? An Exploratory Study." Quality & Safety in Health Care 17 no. 2 (2008): 90-96. doi:10.1136/qshc.2007.023754.

19. Ibid

20. Wolosin, Robert J., Laura Vercler, and Jessica L. Matthews. "Am I Safe Here? Improving Patients' Perceptions of Safety in Hospitals." Journal of Nursing Care Quality 21 no. 1 (2006): 30-8; quiz 39-40.

21. Swayden, Kelli J., Karen K. Anderson, Lynne M. Connelly, Jennifer S. Moran, Joan K. McMahon, and Paul M. Arnold. "Effect of Sitting vs. Standing on Perception of Provider Time at Bedside: A Pilot Study." Patient Education and Counseling 86 no. 2 (2012): 166-171. doi: http://dx.doi.org/10.1016/j.pec.2011.05.024.

22. Millenson, Michael. "Race, Ethnicity, and Patient Engagement." The Health Care Blog, March 7, 2015. http://thehealthcareblog.com/blog/2015/03/07/patient-engagement-ethnicity-and-race/.

23. Ibid

24. Street Jr., Richard L., Howard Gordon, and Paul Haidet. "Physicians' Communication and Perceptions of Patients: Is It How They

Look, How They Talk, or Is It Just the Doctor?" Social Science & Medicine 65 no. 3 (2007): 586-598. doi: http://dx.doi.org/10.1016/j.socscimed.2007.03.036.

25. Alexander, Jeff, Larry Hearld, and Jessica N. Mittler. "Patient-Physician Role Relationships and Patient Activation." Medical Care Research and Review 71 no. 5 (2014): 472-495. doi: 10.1177/1077558714541967.

26. Bucknum, Patrick. "3 Best Practices for Patient Engagement" Hardwired Results 22 (2016): 8. https://www.studergroup.com/hardwired-results/hardwired-results-22/hardwired-results-issue-22-index.

27. Ibid

28. Ibid

29. Whitman, Elizabeth. "Taking Aim at Racial Disparities in Health, Hospitals Put a Shared Decisionmaking Tool to the Test." Modern Healthcare, August 29, 2016. http://www.modernhealthcare.com/article/20160829/NEWS/160829922.

30. Bucknum, Patrick. "3 Best Practices for Patient Engagement" Hardwired Results 22 (2016): 8. https://www.studergroup.com/hardwired-results/hardwired-results-22/hardwired-results-issue-22-index.

31. Amanda Bonser (senior director, Huron Healthcare), in an email to the author based on her notes from attending: Karam, Amelie and Chris Karam. "Millennials to Baby Boomers: Generational Understanding in the Healthcare Workplace." Presentation at Modern Healthcare Women Leaders in Healthcare. Nashville, TN, August 2, 2016.

32. Ibid

33. Ibid

34. Judith Hibbard, in an interview with the author, July 7, 2016.

35. Ibid

36. Ibid

Chapter 7:

1. Sawesi, Suhila, Mohamed Rashrash, Kanitha Phalakornkule, Janet S. Carpenter, and Josette F. Jones. "The Impact of Information Technology on Patient Engagement and Health Behavior Change: A Systematic Review of the Literature." JMIR Medical Informatics 4, no. 1 (2016). doi: 10.2196/medinform.4514

2. JHMCEED. "AMA Health Literacy Video – Short Version." YouTube video, 03:59. Posted August 2012. https://www.youtube.com/watch?v=ubPkdpGHWAQ

3. Baumeister, Roy F., Ellen Bratslavsky, Mark Muraven, and Dianne M. Tice. "Ego Depletion: Is the Active Self a Limited Resource?" Journal of Personality and Social Psychology 74, no. 5 (1998): 1252-1265.

4. Bowerman, Mary. "Children's Hospital Using 'Pokemon GO' to Get Patients Out of Bed." USA Today, July 18, 2016. http://www.usatoday.com/story/tech/nation-now/2016/07/15/motts-childrens-hospital-michigan-pokemon-go-get-children-interacting-rooms-technology/87086698/.

5. Aetna, Inc. "Aetna to Transform Members' Consumer Health Experience Using iPhone, iPad and Apple Watch." Aetna press release, September 27, 2016. http://investor.aetna.com/phoenix.zhtml?c=110617&p=irol-newsarticle&id=2206242, accessed October 5, 2016.

6. McClain, Jasmaine. "Smart Watches, Smart Care: How Wearables Can Improve Patient Engagement." Care Transformation Center Blog, The Advisory Board, May 20, 2016, https://www.advisory.com/Research/Care-Transformation-Center/Care-Transformation-Center-Blog/2016/05/Wearables?WT.mc_id=Email|DailyBriefing+Spotlight|Blog|CTC|2016May31|IT|&elq_cid=1411443&x_id=003C-000001Cd5nxIAB.

7. Ibid

8. Pecci, Alexandra Wilson. "Sharing Notes with Patients Boosts Engagement." HealthLeaders Media, February 19, 2016. http://www.healthleadersmedia.com/sharing-notes-patients-boosts-engagement.

9. Ibid

10. Ibid

11. IHS, Inc. "Global Telehealth Market Set to Expand Tenfold by 2018." IHS Markit press release, January 17, 2014. http://press.ihs.com/press-release/design-supply-chain-media/global-telehealth-market-set-expand-tenfold-2018.

12. Iafolla, Teresa. "36 Telemedicine Statistics You Should Know." eVisit (blog), August 20, 2015. http://blog.evisit.com/36-telemedicine-statistics-know.

13. Stanford Health Care. Emerging Trends in Patient Access. May 9, 2016.

14. Smith, Joe. "Why We're Getting Patient Engagement Backwards." The Health Care Blog, December 4, 2014. http://thehealthcareblog.com/blog/2014/12/04/why-were-getting-patient-engagement-backwards/.

15. Eder, Milton, Sandy G. Smith, James Cappleman, John Hickner, Nancy Elder, and Gurdev Singh. Improving Your Office Testing Process. A Toolkit for Rapid-Cycle Patient Safety and Quality Improvement. Rockville: Agency for Healthcare Research and Quality, 2013. http://www.ahrq.gov/professionals/quality-patient-safety/quality-resources/tools/office-testing-toolkit/officetesting-toolkit7.html#survey

16. Freeman, Harold P. and Rian L. Rodriguez. "History and Principles of Patient Navigation." Cancer 117, no. S15 (2011): 3537-3540. doi: 10.1002/cncr.26262

17. Ibid

18. Ibid

19. Desimini, Esther Muscari, Janine A. Kennedy, Meg F. Helsley, Karen Shiner, Chris Denton, Toni T. Rice, Barbara Stannard, Patrick W. Farrell, Peter A. Marmerstein, and Margaret G. Lewis. "Making the Case for Nurse Navigators." Oncology Issues 26, no. 5 (2011): 26-33.

20. Ibid

21. Richter, Ruthann. "Nationally Renowned Family Physician to Lead Trendsetting Stanford Clinic for Patients with Severe Chronic Disorders." Stanford Medicine press release, October 20, 2011. https://med.stanford.edu/news/all-news/2011/10/nationally-renowned-family-physician-to-lead-trendsetting-stanford-clinic-for-patients-with-severe-chronic-disorders.html

22. Ibid

23. Wasserstein, Paul. "Costs and Outcomes: Does Patient Engagement Work?" Marin Medicine 59, no. 2 (2013) http://www.nbcms.org/about-us/marin-medical-society/magazine/marin-medicine-spring-2013-feature-articles-costs-and-outcomesbrdoes-patient-engagement-work.aspx?pageid=210&tabid=759

24. Ibid

Conclusion:

1. Carman, Kristin L., Pam Dardess, Maureen Maurer, Tom Workman, Deepa Ganachari, and Ela Pathak-Sen. A Roadmap for Patient and Family Engagement in Healthcare Practice and Research. (Prepared by the American Institutes for Research under a grant from the Gordon and Betty Moore Foundation, Dominick Frosch, Project Officer and Fellow; Susan Baade, Program Officer.) Palo Alto: Gordon and Betty Moore Foundation, 2014. www.patientfamilyengagement.org.

ADDITIONAL RESOURCES

ABOUT STUDER GROUP®, A HURON SOLUTION:

A recipient of the 2010 Malcolm Baldrige National Quality Award, Studer Group is an outcomes-based healthcare performance improvement firm that works with healthcare organizations in the United States, Canada, and beyond, teaching them how to achieve, sustain, and accelerate exceptional clinical, operational, and financial results. Working together, we help to get the foundation right so organizations can build a sustainable culture that promotes accountability, fosters innovation, and consistently delivers a great patient experience and the best quality outcomes over time.

To learn more about Studer Group, visit www.studergroup.com/who-we-are/about-studer-group or call 850-439-5839.

STUDER GROUP COACHING:

Studer Group coaches partner with healthcare organizations to create an aligned culture accountable to achieving outcomes together. Working side-by-side, we help to establish, accelerate, and hardwire the necessary changes to create a culture of excellence. This leads to better transparency, higher accountability, and the ability to target and execute specific, objective results that organizations want to achieve.

Studer Group offers coaching based on organizational needs: Evidence-Based Leadership, System Partnership, Specialized Emergency Department, Huron Physician Solutions, and Rural Healthcare.

Learn more about Studer Group coaching by visiting www.studergroup.com/coaching.

STUDER CONFERENCES:

Studer Conferences are exciting interactive learning events that offer a fresh perspective from industry-leading keynote speakers and focused sessions that share evidence-based methods to improve consistency, reduce variance, increase engagement, and create highly profitable organizations. Network with colleagues and experts. Reconnect to your passion for working in healthcare. And do it all while learning new competencies needed to continuously improve the quality and experience of patient-centered care. All Studer Group Conferences offer Continuing Education Credits.

Find out more about upcoming Studer Conferences and register at www.studergroup.com/conferences.

STUDER SPEAKING:

From large association events to exclusive executive training, Studer Group speakers deliver the perfect balance of inspiration and education for every audience. As experienced clinicians and administrators, each speaker has a unique journey to share filled with expertise on a variety of healthcare topics. This personal touch, along with hard-hitting healthcare improvement tactics, empowers your team to take action.

Learn more about Studer Group speaking by visiting www.studergroup.com/speaking.

ABOUT FIRE STARTER PUBLISHING:

Fire Starter Publishing offers intellectual resources for healthcare professionals. We strive to inform healthcare workers of prescriptive to-dos and inspire passion that will encourage action to create change. Our mission is to provide the tools and inspiration to make healthcare better for employees, patients, and physicians.

For over a decade, Fire Starter Publishing has been providing resources to healthcare organizations across the United States, Australia, Canada, China, New Zealand, and Japan. With more than 900,000 publications in circulation, we are a trusted source for proven tactics and tools to help improve employee engagement, build leadership skills, and improve channels of communication.

Explore the Fire Starter Publishing catalog by visiting www.firestarterpublishing.com.

ENGAGEMENT:

Are You Ready for the New Core Competency in Healthcare?

For many years, engagement was considered a "soft" science—something thought about only after addressing the "hard stuff" like volume and reimbursement. Those who buy into this mindset, however, fail to realize the impact engagement actually has on issues such as patient safety, patient perception of care, and, as a result, patient volume and financial performance.

Studer Group has been researching and tracking the impact of employee and physician engagement for over a decade. Our mission as a company—to make healthcare better—commits us to helping healthcare organizations become world-class at engaging leaders, employees, clinicians, and patients and their families.

Everything we do at Studer Group is centered on the understanding that healthcare professionals are values-driven people who want to do work that is purposeful, worthwhile, and makes a difference. In short, they want and need to be fully engaged. That is why results start with engagement. Engagement is the human component of improvement.

When we examine top-performing organizations, we find those that sustain results and maintain high reliability have cultures of high engagement. Through evidence-based tools and tactics, Studer Group helps to build aligned goals, behaviors, and processes that foster an environment that allows people to engage.

Learn more about how Studer Group is helping healthcare organizations build highly engaged cultures at www.studergroup.com/healthcare-engagement.

ABOUT THE AUTHOR

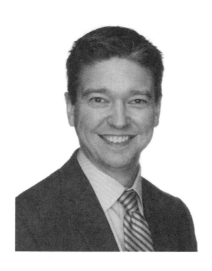

Craig Deao, MHA, has been a member of the senior executive team for Studer Group since 2006. He leads the speaking, conferences, and publishing teams for Studer Group and is also a highly regarded national speaker on topics related to leadership, patient engagement, quality, and patient safety.

In addition to his full-time work with Studer Group, he serves as faculty for the American College of Healthcare Executives.

Since co-leading Studer Group's journey to become a winner of the Malcolm Baldrige Quality Award in 2009, he now spends most weeks inside of healthcare organizations working with boards, medical staffs, and executives to help them architect their own journeys to excellence.

Born and raised in New Orleans, Craig received two bachelor's degrees from Louisiana State University. He received his master's degree in healthcare administration from the University of Minnesota.

Craig now lives in Pensacola, FL, where he serves on the quality committee of his local health system. He has been married to Julie for 11 years, and is the proud father of nine-year-old Sam and six-year-old Jack.

How to Order Additional Copies of

The E-Factor: How Engaged Patients, Clinicians, Leaders, and Employees Will Transform Healthcare

Online:
www.firestarterpublishing.com/e-factor

By phone: 866-354-3473

By mail: Fire Starter Publishing
350 W. Cedar Street, Suite 300
Pensacola, FL 32502

Share this book with your team—and save!
If purchasing for a team to share, please contact Fire Starter Publishing
at 866-354-3473 to learn more about volume savings.